"*Technomorphisms and the Posthuman Turn* is the result of an ongoing collaboration between analysts, inviting the reader to broaden their knowledge from a psychoanalytical vertex and to engage in a critical dialogue toward a posthumanist perspective. We are in the Anthropocene, in which the place of the subject has shifted to the Posthuman era, where the subject is accountable for its acts on the ecosystem. This ontological and epistemological shift encompassing AI and technology directly concerns the human condition, our clinical practice, and theory. Whether deeply versed in the subject or curious novice, this book will challenge, expand, and enrich you. It is a must-read!"

Dr Katy Bogliatto, *IPA Vice-President (2025–2029), Belgian Psychoanalytical Society*

Technomorphisms and the Posthuman Turn

Technomorphisms and the Posthuman Turn explores the profound intersections between psychoanalysis and posthumanism, shedding light on the evolving complexities of subjectivity in a hyper-technological world.

This ground-breaking volume delves into the hybridization of the human, nature, and technology, examining how these intersections reshape notions of gender, sexuality, identity, and subjectivity. Through contributions from leading thinkers, the book addresses the ethical and theoretical challenges posed by posthumanism, including the rise of nomadic subjectivities, prosthetic bodies, and the dominance of digital culture. It critically investigates the impact of these transformations on psychoanalytic theory and practice, urging a re-evaluation of traditional epistemological frameworks. By fostering dialogue with other disciplines, the book seeks to deepen our understanding of unconventional subjectivities and the shifting itineraries of sexuality and gender in contemporary society.

This book is an essential resource for psychoanalysts, scholars, and students interested in the intersections of psychoanalysis, gender studies, posthumanism, and technology. It is also invaluable for anyone seeking to understand the ethical and theoretical implications of living in a world where the boundaries of the human are constantly being redefined.

Leticia Glocer Fiorini, MD, is a training analyst of the Argentine Psychoanalytic Association (APA) and former President of this Society. Overall Chair of the IPA Sexual and Gender Diversity Studies Committee (2021–2025) and Professor of Gender Studies at the University of Buenos Aires, Argentina. She published and gave lectures on femininity and gender and sexual diversity.

Jean Marc Tauszik is a psychoanalyst based in Buenos Aires, Argentina. He is a member of the Caracas Psychoanalytic Society and co-chair for Latin America of the Sexual and Gender Diversity Studies Committee (2021–2025) and chair of the PPL platform (Latin American Psychoanalytic Thought).

Silvia Acosta, PsyD, PhD, is an Argentinian psychoanalyst, member of the SPP and the APC, a member of the IPA Sexual and Gender Diversity Studies Committee (2021–2025), and a co-founder of the FEPAL Working Party on drive constellations and subjectivation processes. She has published psychoanalytic articles and teaches on sexual and gender diversity in Europe and Latin America.

IPA Sexual and Gender Diversity Series
Series Editor: Leticia Glocer Fiorini

Recent titles in the Series include

Polymorphisms
Sexual and Gender Migrations in Contemporary Psychoanalysis
Edited by Leticia Glocer Fiorini, Jean Marc Tauszik, and Silvia Acosta

Gender, Identifications, and Identities
Dialogues at the Edges
Edited by Frances Thomson-Salo, Luca Bruno, and Eva Reichelt

Working Psychoanalytically with Gender Diversity and Sexualities
Resistances to Differences
Edited by Frances Thomson-Salo, Marco Posadas, and Silvia Acosta

Technomorphisms and the Posthuman Turn
A Challenge to Contemporary Psychoanalysis
Edited by Leticia Glocer Fiorini, Jean Marc Tauszik, and Silvia Acosta

Technomorphisms and the Posthuman Turn

A Challenge to Contemporary Psychoanalysis

Edited by
Leticia Glocer Fiorini,
Jean Marc Tauszik, and Silvia Acosta

Routledge
Taylor & Francis Group
LONDON AND NEW YORK

Cover image credit: Getty Images

First published 2027
by Routledge
4 Park Square, Milton Park, Abingdon, Oxon OX14 4RN

and by Routledge
605 Third Avenue, New York, NY 10158

Routledge is an imprint of the Taylor & Francis Group, an informa business

British Library Cataloguing-in-Publication Data
A catalogue record for this book is available from the British Library

ISBN: 978-1-041-32661-8 (hbk)
ISBN: 978-1-041-32660-1 (pbk)
ISBN: 978-1-003-78386-2 (ebk)

DOI: 10.4324/9781003783862

Typeset in Palatino
by Apex CoVantage, LLC

To the authors who contributed with their invaluable thoughts to the subject proposed

Contents

Contributors

Silvia Acosta has a PhD in Psychology and is a psychoanalyst and member of the Asociación Psicoanalítica de Córdoba, Argentina, and the International Psychoanalytic Association (IPA). She currently serves as the Overall Chair of the IPA's Committee on Sexual and Gender Diversity Studies and is the Scientific Secretary of the *International Journal of Psychoanalysis* (IJP) Annual Review in Spanish. She is former Vice President of IPSO for Latin America. As a Professor, she formerly taught the Methodology of Research in the Master's programme in Psychoanalysis at USAL University. Dr. Acosta has directed multiple research programmes subsidized by the IPA, thanks to which she has received the IPA's "Outstanding Contribution to Psychoanalytic Research" and "Training Today" awards.

Rosi Braidotti holds a PhD from the Sorbonne University and is Professor Emeritus at Utrecht University. has devoted herself extensively to researching and writing about feminism, ethics, climate crisis, and post-humanism She is a professor emeritus at Utrecht University and has received significant awards for her academic and humanitarian work. She has received the Humboldt Prize for her career in research and teaching. In 2024, she wrote *Posthumanism, Materialism, Affirmation: Feminist Perspectives*; in 2023 *Affirmative Ethics – the Philosophy of the Big Yes! and How to Live the Anti-Fascist Life*, in a series of Max Weber Lectures at the European University, and *Posthuman Feminism and Affirmative Ethics* in 2019, among many other conferences and published books. Recently, she also published the book "Posthuman Convergence" (2025).

Mónica B. Cragnolini holds a PhD in Philosophy from the University of Buenos Aires, where she is Full Professor of Metaphysics, Special Problems in Metaphysics, and Philosophy of Animality, and Director of the Master's degree in Interdisciplinary Studies of Subjectivity. She is the author of numerous books, including *Nietzsche: Camino y demora* (*Nietzsche: Path and Delay*) (1998); *Moradas nietzscheanas* (*Nietzschean Dwellings*) (2006); *Derrida, un pensador del resto* (*Derrida, A Thinker of the Rest*) (2007); *Extraños animales: filosofía y animalidad en el pensar contemporáneo* (*Strange Animals: Philosophy and Animality in Contemporary*

Thinking) (2016); *¿A quién le importan los animales?* (*Who Cares About Animals?*) (2019); and *Vivir de la sangre de otro: la violencia estructural en el tratamiento de humanos y animales* (*Living Off the Blood of Others: Structural Violence in the Treatment of Humans and Animals*) (2021). She was the winner of the First National Culture Award of the Argentine Republic in Philosophical Essay in 2020.

Helga Fernández practices psychoanalysis. She is a member of the école lacanienne de psychanalyse. She is the editorial director of En el margen, an editorial collective, and editor at Archivida, a publishing house. She is the author of Para un psicoanálisis profano (Archivida, 2020); *La carne humana* (Archivida, 2022; Mexico, 2023); *Mandíbulas autómatas* (En el margen, 2024); *La hiperstición, la más nueva de las letosas* (En el margen, 2024); *Entre la lumbre y la penumbra* (Cielo invertido, 2025); *La función del amigo. Una tensión deseante* (En el margen, 2026); and *Reír hasta caer. 22 vueltas y un tropezón alrededor del chiste en Macedonio Fernández* (Lirio, 2026). Forthcoming: *El psicoanálisis en cuestión* (Nocturna editorial).

Francesca Ferrando is Professor of Philosophy at NYU Liberal Studies, New York University. She is a leading voice in the field of posthuman studies and the founder of the Global Posthuman Network. She has received numerous honours and awards, including the Sainati Prize with the Recognition of the President of Italy. She has published extensively on these topics; her latest book is *Philosophical Posthumanism* (2019). In the history of TED talks, she was the first speaker to give a talk on the subject of posthuman. The American magazine "Origins" included her among the 100 people who are changing the world. For more information: http://www.theposthuman.org/.

Leticia Glocer Fiorini is a psychoanalyst in the teaching function of the Argentine Psychoanalytic Association and holds a master's degree in Psychoanalysis from USAL University. She is a Professor of the Master's degree in "Interdisciplinary Studies of Subjectivity" (University of Buenos Aires) and Overall Chair of the Sexual and Gender Diversity Studies Committee of the International Psychoanalytical Association (2021–2025). A Past President of the Argentine Psychoanalytic Association, she is also the former Chair of the Publications Committees for both the IPA and the APA. Her authored books include *Lo femenino y el pensamiento complejo* (2001, 2nd ed. 2020), published in English as *Deconstructing the Feminine* (2007, 2nd ed. 2024); and *La diferencia sexual en debate* (2015), published in English as *Sexual Difference in Debate* (2017). She has published extensively on femininity, sexual and gender diversity, and unconventional parenting. She received the Cárcamo Award from the Argentine Psychoanalytic Association and was awarded with the Konex Prize in Psychoanalysis, 2026.

Mariano Horenstein is a psychoanalyst with teaching function (APC/FEPAL/IPA) and served as a Representative for Latin America on the IPA Board. He is the former Editor-in-Chief of *Calibán-Revista Latinoamericana de Psicoanálisis* and Member of the "Geographies of Psychoanalysis" research group. His published books include Artists, Writers and Philosophers on Psychoanalysis. From the Couch, Routledge (2025); *The Compass and the Couch, Mimesis* (2018); *Funambulistas. Travesía adolescente y riesgo, Viento de Fondo* (2020); *Psicoanálisis en lengua menor, Viento de Fondo* (2016); *De que falamos quando falamos de psicanálise? Conferencias gaúchas, Artes & Ecos* (2026). His work has been recognized with the E. Hayman, FEPAL, Lucian Freud, and Garma international awards, among others. Further information: www.marianohorenstein.com

Victor J. Krebs holds a PhD in Philosophy from the University of Notre Dame and is a professor at PUCP. He is the author of *Del alma y el arte* (1997), *La recuperación del sentido* (2007), *La imaginación pornográfica* (2017), and *Human Virtuality and Digital Life* (2022), the latter of which received the Gradiva and Courage to Dream (APA) awards. As the Coordinator of the Latin American Network of Posthumanism, his work integrates philosophy, psychoanalysis, aesthetics, and posthumanism. He is currently writing *Dreaming Life in the Digital Age* and *A Guide for the Poor Hedonist.*

Helena Maldonado Goti is a Mexican psychoanalyst and member of the École Lacanienne de Psychanalyse (ELP, where she also serves as the Director of the ELP's *e-dicciones Justine* project, and practices psychoanalysis in Mexico City. She studied psychology at the Faculty of Psychology at UNAM and obtained both her master's degree and PhD in philosophy at the Faculty of Philosophy and Letters from the same institution. She has taught philosophy in master's and doctoral programmes in Psychoanalysis. Her publications can be found on the *e-dicciones Justine* website. She has also published in the magazine *Me Cayó el Veinte* and in the *Philosophy Journal of the Ibero-American University.*

Patricia Porchat is Professor of Psychology at UNESP, Brazil. She held the *Chaire genre* in 2022, offered by GIS Institut du Genre in collaboration with Université Paris Cité. She coordinates the Postgraduate programme in Sexual Education at UNESP and post-doctorate at Paris Diderot University following her Doctorate in Clinical Psychology (USP). She is a researcher at the Center for Human Rights and Health of the LGBT Population (NUDHES) of the Faculty of Medical Sciences at Santa Casa de São Paulo. Her books include *Freud and the Reality Test* (2005) and *Psychoanalysis and Transsexualism: Deconstructing Genders and Pathologies with Judith Butler* (2014); she is also the co-organizer of the book *Psychoanalysis and Gender: Feminist and Queer Narratives in Brazil and Argentina* (2018).

María Luisa Silva Checa is a psychoanalyst in the teaching function of the Peruvian Society of Psychoanalysis. She is a Clinical Psychologist and holds a master's degree in Theoretical Studies in Psychoanalysis from the Pontifical Catholic University of Peru (PUCP). She is Professor in the master's programme at PUCP and the SPP Institute, Member of the board of the Latin American Encounters on Winnicott's Thought, and is the editor of the book *Tejiendo ideas y sensibilidades* (*Weaving Ideas and Sensibilities*) (2024). She is the Editor-in-chief of *Calibán, FEPAL Magazine*. She was the winner of the FEPAL Award 2014.

Jean Marc Tauszik is a member of the Caracas Psychoanalytic Society (SPC). He served as the Vice President and Scientific Secretary of OCAL from 2010 to 2012 and 2012 to 2014, respectively. He is the current Chair of Latin American Psychoanalytic Thought (PPL) and was Co-Chair of APA Psychoanalytic Colloquiums. He was a member of the IPA Committee on Gender and Sexual Diversity from 2017 to 2021 and former Co-Chair for Latin America (2021–2025). He co-edited (together with Fernando Gómez) *Contemporary Latin American Psychoanalysis*, Volume I (2018). In 2009, he received the award of the International Psychoanalytic Studies Organization (IPSO).

Series Preface

Leticia Glocer Fiorini

With this volume we continue to publish the *Sexual and Gender Diversity Series* edited by the S&GDS Committee. The aim of the series' project is to explore, expand, and update psychoanalytic thoughts focusing on today's sexual and gender migrations. This objective is part of the Committee's mandate to present debates and controversies in psychoanalysis in order to better understand contemporary changes to subjectivities.

This applies to the review of epistemological, theoretical, and clinical tools in the psychoanalytical field focusing on changes which demand continuing to develop new concepts and to reconsider others. By confronting them, we might find agreements and disagreements which should be worked through in an open dialogue. In this frame, our perspective is to grasp a contemporary and present point of view on these topics. At the same time, there are crucial axes of psychoanalysis, from Freud's onwards, that should be maintained.

There is a complex fabric which includes different psychoanalytic theories, different clinical approaches, as well as different cultures in the same or diverse latitudes. Certainly, the necessary intersection between psychic reality with otherness and culture runs throughout this proposal.

All these facts lead to set out relevant ideas and themes that were and are discussed by several psychoanalytic theories, as well as by gender and post-gender theories. This approach inevitably includes the clarification of the logical and epistemic perspectives from which different proposals are read today. Listening to other viewpoints inevitably guides us to a better listening of our patients, especially of what is new and original – meaning a space of freedom both to analysts and to patients.

In this context, not only concordances can be found, but also divergences that should be sustained in tension in the perspective of exploring which are the effects of the crucial changes that are part of current societies. Indeed, this implies extra work for the reader to illuminate these contradictions in a fruitful way. In this way, our purpose has been to go beyond a unique, uniform line of thought in order to sustain differences which each reader might process creatively, and surpass as well.

The S&GDS Committee's objective is to share these ideas with the psychoanalytic community and with professionals of other disciplines, with the aim of generating a productive interchange between the text and the reader. We assume the challenge of displaying these debates that involve significant contributions to think about contemporary construction of subjectivity.

Our special acknowledgement goes to the authors for their outstanding contributions, to the International Psychoanalytic Association for their support to undertake this project, and to Stefano Bolognini, past president of the IPA, who created the S&GDS Committee in 2017.

Lastly, we acknowledge the Committee's members for their commitment to organizing dialogues, conferences, and study days in Europe, North America, and South America that inspired us to edit this series focused on sexual and gender diversity.

IPA Sexual and Gender Diversity Studies Committee
Leticia Glocer Fiorini, Series Editor

Introduction

Leticia Glocer Fiorini, Jean Marc Tauszik, and Silvia Acosta

This book is inspired by the Second Latin American Dialogue of the Sexual and Gender Diversity Studies Committee of the International Psychoanalytic Association (IPA) that took place on June 4–5, 2021. Its title, *Technomorphisms and the Posthuman Turn: A Challenge to Contemporary Psychoanalysis,* is in line with our first Dialogue, *Polymorphisms: Sexual and Gender Migrations in Contemporary Psychoanalysis*, developed in 2019 in Buenos Aires and published by Routledge in 2025.

On this occasion, we had decided to expand the notion of gender and sexual diversity, deploying an interplay with new perspectives on the human condition that include multiple, heterogeneous, and dynamic ways of conceiving subjectivities and its relations with nature, biotechnology, and cyber-technology, which make us inhabitants of multiple and complex universes. These hybridizations between the human, the eco-environment, and technology impact on the construction of subjectivity and the notions of identity, and they have ethical implications as it is not possible to conceive them in isolation from the other components of our planet. The posthuman perspective challenges us to revise our theory, beliefs, and biases on current subjectivities.

In other words, our research on sexual and gender migrations is situated in a cultural, social, and hyper-technological context where the attack on life and the planet is having a full impact on present-day subjectivities. The extinction of human life is no longer just a fantasy. Posthumanism is present and must be investigated in order to be included in our theorizations and clinical work.

Psychoanalysis is no stranger to these changes: we are in the presence of ontological changes that have an impact on our theoretical approach to the subject and subjectivity; our epistemological bases demand revisions and expansions that require us to focus on intersections with other disciplines, and they challenge fixed and eternal definitions about the determinants of psychic structuring.

The intersection between psychoanalysis and posthumanism opens crucial lines to investigate the construction of subjectivity and its complexity,

DOI: 10.4324/9781003783862-1

as well as the dualistic thinking of modernity and its ethical drifts. Here, too, a politics of psychoanalysis is present that demands to be investigated.

Today's societies are in fact facing changes that have no return:

- Nomadic subjectivities, the achieved identity of which is an ideal that is never reached.
- Prosthetic, intervened bodies.
- A digital culture that replaces, complements, and at times sweeps away literate culture. It implies a reflection on current definitions of the modes of psychic inscription, representation, unrepresentable, unrepresented.
- A structural limitation of our technique to the point that, in some theoretical spaces within psychoanalysis, the logic of "looking for the best technical device for the widest symbolic access to subjective productions" has been inverted by "whether or not we let the human experience enter by perforating the limits of our frame".

Each aspect implies not only a theoretical but also an ethical debate on which psychoanalysis takes different positions that define in what sense it can or cannot start a conversation in a shared framework with posthumanism.

How these changes impact on the psychoanalytic discipline and on psychoanalysts themselves is part of the reflections included in this volume.

Our daily clinic is the scenario where these changes and processes take place; theories are today revising their positions. Our objective was to establish a dialogue with other analysts who work with these concerns, as well as with recognized representatives of other related disciplines in order to achieve higher levels of criticism and new constructions.

The Editors
Leticia Glocer Fiorini, Overall Chair 2021–2025
Jean Marc Tauszik, Co-Chair for Latin America 2021–2025
Silvia Acosta, Overall Chair 2025–2029
Sexual and Gender Diversity Studies Committee of the IPA

Part 1

Posthuman Feminism

1 Posthuman Feminism[1]

Sexuality Beyond Gender

Rosi Braidotti

Dear friends from Buenos Aires,
Dear Leticia Glocer Fiorini,

I wish I could be there in person; it's been a long time since I've visited that beloved city. Argentina is so close to my family history, so close to my heart. I wish we could have this conversation face to face; maybe someday we can meet.

Congratulations for this wonderful meeting "Technomorphisms and the posthuman turn" (2021), on posthumanism.

I would like to participate in this meeting by referring especially to notions such as psychoanalysis, affectivity, sexuality, and gender – all topics very close to our hearts.

It is difficult to listen to a talk for too long, so I will try to be concise and concise. I will do my best to fit it into the proceedings as if I were there.

If you know anything about my ideas, you will know that I do not define posthumanism as a point in the future, not as a cyborg utopia, not as a transhumanist process of improving man to become more machine-like.

I see posthumanism as a feature of our historical context, and I understand posthumanist critical thinking as an intervention on central discussions on posthumanist predicaments.

This is a very different starting position, very immanent, incarnated, where we are in a posthuman convergence, very involved in very advanced technological developments on the one hand, and in an acceleration of the process of environmental devastation, even species extinction, on the other.

We are in a simultaneity of very opposite effects: we are landing vehicles on Mars to explore for water and minerals, possibilities of life, while life on this planet is threatened by so many factors related to "extractionist" economies, empty, environmentally ruthless models that promote resistant patterns of racism, sexism, ecocide, and disregard and indifference towards the materiality of our living environment.

So the posthuman convergence is a "crash" of very different and opposite effects that are accelerating in front of our eyes; not a utopia about the future, not something a Hollywood movie is showing, but something that is already here.

DOI: 10.4324/9781003783862-3

The mutation of the state of the human is happening right now. Looking at the situation in which we are involved, it is an example of this: the pandemic of COVID-19, which prevents us from being together today holding this conversation in person, is the human disaster *par excellence*, produced by the violent interference in the ecological balance of the coexistence of multiple species. This pandemic is at the heart of the environmental problem, of the socioeconomic problem, of all these concerns.

And paradoxically, this contingency has resulted in the increased use of technology and all its digital mediations increasing the hope in finding vaccines and biomedical solutions; intensifying human dependence on a super-technified economy known as cognitive capitalism – I will come back to this concept – in a greater dependence on highly advanced technology and that technological model of growth which is the source of the problem in the first place.

The pandemic can exemplify the interconnectedness of the human and non-human assembled in the development of multiple ecologies that structure our existence. Environmental ecology, socioeconomic ecology, affective, emotional, and psychic ecologies – psychoanalysis has to be part of this conversation – illustrate our dependence on all of them and also, paradoxically, increase our dependence on super-advanced technologies that are at the heart of advanced capitalism and are at the heart of the problem in the first place.

The contradiction is exciting and it is also totally infuriating. Totally full of promise and absolutely full of despair. And I want to start from here, from this specific affective economy. The affects we surround ourselves with, alternations of complex and contradictory emotions, which for me are typical of the posthuman convergence.

An intense sense of suffering, the loss of more than three million lives, in addition to the non-human ones, the sense of increased vulnerability, the lack of hope, and at the same time the desire for the future as well, are present.

Four industrial revolutions and six extinctions had happened. The humanistic notion of progress has been moving away from the enormous amount of evidence of the failure or flaws of the growth model. The increased sense of mortality, the proximity of death and extinction, go hand in hand with fantasies of immortality or transhumanist delusions of grandeur: more than human, even superhuman, through technological enhancement.

I think that the alternating balance of affects or emotions is something to be taken with extreme seriousness. I have mentioned transhumanism twice so far. Let me clarify this:

There is a notion of transhumanism, which is the conventional and dominant form of posthumanist practice. It is the notion you will find in Silicon Valley, which claims that man and computer can be merged; it is the old California hippie idea that human consciousness could be uploaded into a computer, behind movies like *The Matrix*, which exalt illusions that man can be enhanced through machines.

But there is also, more seriously, the hard core of academic transhumanism, which has one of its great centres at Oxford University, with Nick Bostrom (2018) and his team of brilliant scientists who argue that our brain, human thinking capacity, is being decried by the computational networks that we have already created, that, consequently, human intelligence needs to be enhanced by increased interaction with technology, and that there are neural enhancements, through different forms of implants, through different forms of intimate connections with technology. This is a serious research project, funded with millions of dollars by Oxford University for the future of humanity. It is a project called "Superintelligence", and it is a project about the improvement of the human being developed in the name of humanity, in the name of scientific development, in the name of a noble and rigorous rational research.

This type of project is in line with the heart of the posthumanist message, the transhumanist message, in the sense of affirming that we need man to be improved in order to achieve the speed of technological development.

We are here facing a reduction of the concept of "intelligence" understood as "speed" (of processing), in a reduction of "humanity" to "thinking capacity", and we have a reduction of "thinking capacity" to a Cartesian model of an intelligence based on the mind, separated from the body. So, it is a very traditional "soon-humanist" model of high-tech work.

In critical posthumanism, from where I – and many others – think, it is a critique of this; it is a way of saying "you cannot reduce the notion of mind or thinking capacity to these factors". It is a return even to a pre-Cartesian era; it is even prior to what Freud taught us when he said that thought is something that one does with one's whole organism. It predates even some developments within qualitative neuroscience – I am thinking of the work of Antonio Damasio (2010) or Andy Clark (2011) on distributive consciousness – before these qualitative neuroscientists proved the point that affectivity, desire, and emotions are substantial cognitive tools that involve the whole body. And that, in fact, the body is an extended surface, related to multiple human and non-human sources. Some of these sources are technological but many are simply environmental, social, and psychic sources. You cannot think if you do not have basic needs such as fresh air, clean water, a roof over your head, and other basic facilities.

Thought is the "endowment" of the world; posthumanist materialism holds this clearly: we think with the rest of the world.

So posthumanism is an intervention on dominant forms of transhumanism which represent advanced forms of capitalism. I think what we see, in this pandemic, with the struggles over vaccines, when you see the huge economic disparities, where you also see increased death rates because of increased poverty, or disadvantages in racialized communities relative to conventional white communities.

Viruses do not invent injustices, but they certainly highlight them, put them on **the map: the difficulties**, the complications of this moment, and the acceptance that humanity really will be affected in a number of operations about what today constitutes the sources of capital gains, the sources of life, the sources of valuable supplies, and the sources of capitalization or profit.

So, I would like then to lay the foundations of our exercise: that is here we are, in the middle of this pandemic, forced to be mediated by the screen, forced to have to see ourselves in this picture, assuming that thinking is something that happens to me "from here to here", disconnected from everything. When in fact my arguments go in the opposite direction.

Asserting that we need to think in an embodied way, inserted in affective relations of assembled subjectivities. Posthumanism, in this sense, is materialistic, about heterogeneous relations between human and non-human elements assembled with strong vital elements in them.

The vital elements materialized in my work lead me back to the French continental tradition of "Bodily" materialism, carnal materialism, thinking of the body when it is not reduced to a biological unit; the body is a heterogeneous assembly of human and non-human elements, of environmental, social, and affective elements; relational and, consequently, negotiable in process (but not fluid in any relativistic sense of the term).

Elementally rooted basic elements in the earth, water and indispensable oxygen, also technologically mediated, inspire all the affections and passions we have and motivate our species and cultures forever.

Over time I have become more and more in a "Deleuzian spinosismo" in the sense of thinking in an "ontological desire" to perceive that our existence is what makes us human, is what makes us being; the species that we are: *conatos*, potency, the desire to go on, being, enjoying the simplicity and the complexity of being alive.

Everything that it means to be alive should be perceived in our existence, even when it comes to ways of dying. In fact, death as part of the process of life and even the discussion about impersonal death or personal death are issues that are part of the "contract" of being alive. Death as part of an ongoing process is proper to being a corporeally and affectively related and embodied material entity.

The central issue in this discussion is the issue of language. The long legacy of psychoanalysis is one of the unfortunate situations with the great popularity of Deleuze and Guattari's (1987) materialism that cannot be misunderstood. Psychoanalysis is not a discussion about whether Lacan (2006) was wrong or Freud (1920/1955), (1923/1961) was wrong. Materialism has thrown psychoanalysis out of the window; it has denied something about a specific form, a goal of life that we have obtained from psychoanalysis. So, I think we need to correct this, because there is no Deleuze or Guattari (1983) without psychoanalysis. *The theory of affects close to materialism emerges from the long legacy of psychoanalysis as a philosophy of desire, a material understanding of the body as a machine of desire – not from any technical or terminological reductionism, but as a number of elements related instinctively – a difficult word – to desire, to being alive. Even the death instinct, in the Freudian machine, is a part of a mechanism of the generation of a desire to persevere, to go forward.*

So, what language to use?

How to frame the affectivity of the time we are in?

It is one of our great concerns, particularly in times of such intense collective loss. These are times of mourning, times of compassion, of general global care – a time of deep reflection not only on our mortality and vulnerability but also on the achievements and results of collective efforts to develop, to create general welfare, and to have technological development. How do we frame this?

I think that sensitivity to language, a kind of care about how we nominate, is something we have to go back to, not only in our academic discussions but also in public discourse where the levels of dialogue have become tremendously destructive. Everything is dichotomized, everything is weaponized, and everything is reduced to being for or against, in a completely simplified way. Complexity seems to have a very hard life these days; complexity is everything that philosophy, literature, and critical theory are concerned with.

The opposite of complexity is not simplicity; that would be too simple. The opposite of complexity is simplification; nowadays everything must be simplified to the point of extreme stupidity. And we must not avoid facing this, in such intense times of posthuman development. We must return to a collective respect for complexity, in accordance with language, for the "happiness of expression" as Virginia Woolf (2002) liked to say, to enable us to do justice to the challenges around us.

I believe that all this is part of the legacy of the psychoanalytic tradition where language is not only in a sense of communication, where language is the ontological side of the constitution of our subjectivity, but it is where we recognize ourselves and relate to each other.

We must return to this because of the complexity of language and the understanding that there are rules by which we are related on a conscious and unconscious level, where the unconscious is a flowing affect that connects us and that is not capable of being controlled by reason, where it is not possible to think of a "supra-consciousness" that supervises all that we are.

Affective desire, as materially embodied, is explored through post-psychoanalytic readings on subjectivity understood in a relational sense where we are linked among humans but also with non-human factors such as the multiple ecologies that Guattari (2014) brings, as well as Maturana (1998), Varela (2017), and other thinkers who develop on environmental, affective, social and psychic complexities. Even the perfect simplicity without simplification is complex.

A couple more rules regarding the posthuman must be approached with caution. There is no single way to position oneself within the tradition of critical posthumanism, as there is an understanding that "man" was never a neutral category to which one could ascribe.

"Human" is a category laden with power relations and rights; it is a way of generating concrete hierarchical distinctions between different degrees of humanity. Through the sexualization of the other (women and LGBTQ+ groups), the racialization of the other (Black people, Indigenous peoples, and non-Europeans), and the naturalization of the other (animals, plants, and the planet), they are excluded from the category of "full humanity".

In fact, "being human" is a great privilege, a category with significant control and restrictions; it is a very specific, very particular representation of reality, where "man" is male, white, *a priori* heterosexual, living with his wife and children in an urban area, speaking a standardized language, a citizen who enjoys a welfare state and legal security.

I am paraphrasing here not only postcolonial feminism, but also Viveiros de Castro (2015) and what Deleuze and Guattari (1987) understand as the concept of "man", where "human" is the colonization of the human. My struggle is with European humanism as an ideology of conquest and exclusion; at the same time, it is a sequence of beliefs in science, technology, and reason that allow us to carry that forward and be what we are today.

One of the things on my mind today is a major undertaking currently underway in the exploration of Mars and space, through NASA and other actors seeking other forms of life, but also minerals and new sources of well-being. In fact, it is interesting to note that this space of exploration is today a private initiative; 80% of exploration is in private hands, such as those of Elon Musk, Richard Branson of Virgin, or Jeff Bezos of Amazon.

These individuals receive contracts from NASA; the most recent was awarded to Elon Musk in 2021, through which they are driving the space industry. Musk plans to produce the spacecraft and vehicles to land on the Moon with a human crew by 2025 or 2026. One might think of this, if they wish, as science fiction, but it isn't. It is the world we live in now.

Mars exploration is happening now, but what we need to understand is that it is a private enterprise. It is not focused on the world; it is not the Cold War between America and the Soviet Union – it is private. With money, with NASA of course, in its competition with Chinese ambitions – that is true. But it is privatized. And if you listen to what Elon Musk or Jeff Bezos have to say about it, the discourse is pure transhumanism.

Elon Musk has said that we must leave Earth because its resources are exhausted. The planet is depleted; we have to go to another planet to ensure that humans have enough resources to continue living as we have lived until now. To continue overproducing and dumping waste, amidst tremendous structural inequality – pure transhumanism. Earth is finished; off to Mars we go.

In fact, and to make it clearer, NASA astronauts have the image of the Vitruvian Man printed on their suits.

Leonardo da Vinci's representation of the humanist man is the symbol of our space exploration. Because transhumanism is the exaltation of humanism, they believe in man – but in that man, the very man whom critical posthumanism calls into question. I'm not saying anything about it; I'm just reading the world we live in, the way things happen.

In a world structured this way, we must truly understand that the human is not a neutral category. It is a category laden with power, rights, and exclusion. And again, feminist theory, race theory, and Indigenous and Black philosophies have been saying this for decades. If humanism is not neutral, posthumanism cannot be neutral.

There are many ways to be posthumanist. And my view is that depending on how we understand the emergencies around us – for example, the ongoing struggles against inequalities, injustices, racism, sexism, ecocide, all of them – and the way those situations are linked to recent developments in high technology, it might seem like we can wait; it might look like something not so urgent.

And I ask you to think again because we are in an urgent race not only in terms of the health of our planet, of our planet's resources, but of ourselves, of our own health or our own resources. People are exhausted.

The future seems to be disappearing from our horizon. Everything seems to be closing in, fading away. A sense of impossibility is taking hold of our students very strongly, and when this feeling of sadness, of helplessness, of impossibility takes root in our souls, then we are in real trouble.

I truly agree with Deleuze and Guattari (1983), who define this as a form of micro-fascism – this sense of impossibility, that there is nothing left to strive for, that the horizon is closing in on us.

Therefore, the social construction of a horizon of hope is of central importance. We must work to create affirmations, affections, and projects that can collectively build a sense of hope.

Thus, posthumanism is not the denial of suffering, not the denial of injustices; it is a way of reworking them, based on a relational materialist philosophy growing out of a critical reading of Spinoza (2005), Deleuze and Guattari (1987), from feminism, from Viveiros de Castro (2015), and from Indigenous philosophies – where it is extremely important to place a vote of confidence in the elemental materiality of our planet and our context, directed from the multiple ecologies to which we belong toward a sense of purpose, a sense of the necessity for a social construction of hope before it is too late.

It is urgent; it is not, therefore, an optional extra. If one looks at the general policy of transhumanism, NASA has announced, and the European Space Agency has announced, that they will be sending women, people of color, or even people with disabilities – those deemed "desirable" – into space as part of the space program, which means we will have an intergalactic program with equal opportunities for access to the program. Which is fine; it is part of the human tradition that we achieve emancipation, and we will be sending minorities into the world of the future as well.

But for some of us, for some on our planet Earth, for our immanent, embodied, relational, and affective condition, here and now, the sense of being part of this, the politics of this planetary location compels me to look closely and urgently speak out about these peculiar economic policies of sacrifice.

There are people who are willing to give up, to give up the entire planet by saying "Mars is better"; there are people willing to give up "sections" of the planet – dehumanization that excludes others whose lives do not matter, disposable bodies that can be left to die.

Look at what happened with the vaccine war during the pandemic and the way public health seems to have transformed into this humanitarian emergency – in a certain sense, a deadly one – no matter the cost.

It is urgent to intervene in this political economy that is not only a biopolitics but also a necropolitics, where we all live to die, to let die.

Foucault (1998), one of my mentors, said – and as I state very clearly in some of my classes – that biopolitics is not about how to live longer, but about who lives, regardless of what must be authorized or allowed to die. Only death, in an extinction of the human and non-human on a scale we have never seen before.

I believe this is urgent, and I believe that posthumanism is not a luxury problem we can put off until later; it is an urgent problem concerning intervention in the acceleration of capital, the acceleration of industrial production, the acceleration of the Earth's death, the acceleration of the sixth extinction, anthropocentrism – centered on capital – totally controlled by people who have never considered themselves fully human.

My critical posthumanism (Braidotti, 2020) is a vision of the future that emerges from those who were never the "man of reason", as Genevieve Lloyd (1984) pointed out – a man who was never the reason for this – those who were always marginalized. We have a vision of the future and the present rooted in the tradition of science fiction feminism and Afrofuturism; minorities are visions of the future, but more importantly, we are concerned with the present.

It is this idea of posthuman subjectivity, this notion of embodied relational and affective humanity – in my case, built upon my early thoughts on nomadic subjectivity (Braidotti, 2018). It is a heterogeneous, relational subjectivity; it involves the human and the non-human; it is negotiable; it is an ontology of becoming, of the advent of being in process, guided by an ontological notion of desire – that fundamental passion that reveals to us all that persists in existence. It has significant implications, of course, for a vision of sexuality.

Working from a materialist perspective of Deleuze (2001) and Spinoza (2005), I have always said that one of the keys to posthuman critical thought is sexuality before, with, and beyond gender. Sexuality as an elemental human and non-human force.

It encompasses what I call the sexed nature of matter. It is a very interesting concept that asserts that sexuality is never a neutral element; it is not;

it operates in other species, in animals, in insects. Everything that lives is sexed.

The sexed is not the gender system; sexuality is not masculine or feminine.

The gender system is a binary mechanism that allows us to grasp the immanent complexity of living organisms. The sexed is there before any form of intervention by our systems of social coding.

It is not gender that creates sexes; that is incorrect. I have argued this for years: sexuality is an elemental force of animate matter, in all species. And that is where psychoanalysis is incredibly important. Even beyond the non-human, singular aspects of human sexuality, of the condition of being sexual; or being part of a life cycle of life and death, which connects us to countless other species.

Reconnecting with sexuality beyond gender, liberating the sexual desire of all living things, is a way to dismantle the gender system that separates us in so many ways and generates so much pressure.

And also to rediscover a way of understanding vital forces, desire, and passion beyond binaries; the binary sex–gender system is truly unnecessary for understanding complexity as the principle of NOT ONE. It is not univocal, but a multiplicity of ways of differing not only from the patriarchal binary categorical system, but within each category itself.

Multiple degrees of difference. Across the rainbow of LGBTQ+ variations, but also within the total spectrum of human and non-human possibilities.

It implies that sexuality is the joyful tendency of all living organisms to persevere in existence and to enjoy the fact of being able to insist on persevering. One can infer from this perspective the profound optimism of Spinoza's ideas (2005): *conatus*, all that is living, enjoying, persevering in existence.

Many people may feel irritated by this Spinozian perspective, or, with reference to Deleuze (2001), may consider his idea of "persevering in existence" to be *naive* and uncritical, but then open your eyes, look at life as it lives, beyond the anthropocentric gaze, look at the mechanical sense of the self-replication of living beings and the simple enjoyment of it.

Some people may believe there is something mystical in this perspective; that is not my case. I remain deeply secular, but by recombining ourselves, reattaching ourselves to the elemental path of sexed matter, through infinite forms of becoming, traversing all categories, into thousands of small sexes, through thousands of small variations of being sexed matter, of the way the sexed expresses itself in a posthuman world, I find in this one of the most enjoyable, most exciting things, with the most challenging perspectives.

Posthuman sexuality lies beyond gender, in a multiplicity of possible experiences, multiple ways of being men, women, and everything in between. It must be one of the most exciting moments in the history of gender relations.

Of course, this does not happen in a vacuum; it happens within cognitive capitalism. Cognitive capitalism is a system of profits (gains) based on knowledge of everything we experience. Knowledge about hormones, about chromosomes, about neural systems, about algorithms and computational systems – all of this is part of contemporary gender.

Technologies – gender technologies – that produce the entire business of pleasure, constituting a profitable machinery that we are witnessing. I believe a posthuman approach to all this is very stoic. Very sober; it involves distancing oneself from the blatant manipulation and commodification of sexuality.

The example I have in mind is Gwyneth Paltrow selling candles that smell like her vagina – please, I'm busy. Or creating a gender-porn industry right before our eyes. Thinking about sexuality beyond gender is a way to break away from this and say no, thank you.

Taking a step back, reflecting on what the matter of sexed matter means, connected to other equally sexed organisms in this deeply embodied materialism – which I believe is one of the greatest, most intelligent moments of this difficult era.

Sexuality beyond gender, sexuality as the ontology of desire, embodied and engaged relationally and affectively. This is the philosophical backdrop of a critical posthumanism that looks at the transhumanist delusion (the illusion) and asks: where are our bodies, where are the elements embedded in our environment, where are the others – the sexed, racialized, naturalized others considered less than the "man" of reason?

What does the future look like if you are never fully human? Can we even design possible futures? Look at the work done in disability studies, one of the incredible fields where the greatest discoveries can be made, where other bodies can be designed, working on others, relating others with different capabilities. Multiple ways of negotiating what a human can become.

And within this vast focus of attention, for those who are not considered fully human – the dehumanized, the non-human others – let's see what we can say about what the future looks like.

Not just to send ourselves into outer space, but by remembering that, right now, as we care for a damaged planet during a difficult time for us, we can recall that the human is not neutral; we are not all equal; we differ in so many ways, but one of the most challenging paradoxes of these posthuman convergences is that at this particular point in time, we are in this together, and we are the only ones who cannot get out of this problem together.

It is time to rebuild that heterogeneous "us" – internally differentiated, embodied, and relationally and affectively engaged: that we are not equal but that we are united in this.

I wish you all the best; the truth is, I miss you. All the best – take care, stay healthy, keep up the good work, and best wishes to everyone.

Thanks.

Note

1 Lecture given by R. Braidotti for the Dialogue "Technomorphisms: The posthuman turn and contemporary psychoanalysis", organized by the IPA's Sexual and Gender Diversity Studies Committee, Buenos Aires, December 2021.

References

Bostrom, N. (2018). *Superintelligence: Paths, dangers, strategies*. Oxford University Press. (Original work published 2014)

Braidotti, R. (2018). *The posthuman*. Polity Press. (Original work published 2013)

Braidotti, R. (2020). *Posthuman knowledge*. Polity Press. (Original work published 2019)

Clark, A. (2011). *Supersizing the mind: Embodiment, action, and cognitive extension*. Oxford University Press. (Original work published 2008)

Damasio, A. (2010). *The feeling of what happens: Body and emotion in the making of consciousness*. Mariner Books. (Original work published 1999)

Deleuze, G. (2001). *Spinoza: Practical philosophy* (R. Hurley, Trans.). City Lights. (Original work published 1970)

Deleuze, G., & Guattari, F. (1983). *Anti-Oedipus: Capitalism and schizophrenia* (R. Hurley, M. Seem, & H. R. Lane, Trans.). University of Minnesota Press. (Original work published 1972)

Deleuze, G., & Guattari, F. (1987). *A thousand plateaus: Capitalism and schizophrenia* (B. Massumi, Trans.). University of Minnesota Press. (Original work published 1980)

Foucault, M. (1998). *The history of sexuality: Vol. 1: An introduction* (R. Hurley, Trans.). Penguin Classics. (Original work published 1976)

Freud, S. (1920/1955). *Beyond the pleasure principle*. In J. Strachey (Ed. & Trans.), *The standard edition of the complete psychological works of Sigmund Freud* (Vol. 18, pp. 1–64). Hogarth Press.

Freud, S. (1923/1961). *The ego and the id*. In J. Strachey (Ed. & Trans.), *The standard edition of the complete psychological works of Sigmund Freud* (Vol. 19, pp. 1–66). Hogarth Press.

Guattari, F. (2014). *The three ecologies* (I. Pindar & P. Sutton, Trans.). Bloomsbury Academic. (Original work published 1989)

Lacan, J. (2006). *Écrits* (B. Fink, Trans.). W. W. Norton. (Original work published 1966)

Lloyd, G. (1984). *The man of reason: "Male" and "female" in Western philosophy*. University of Minnesota Press.

Maturana, H. R., & Varela, F. J. (1998). *The tree of knowledge: The biological roots of human understanding*. Shambhala. (Original work published 1987)

Spinoza, B. (2005). *Ethics* (E. Curley, Trans.). Penguin Classics. (Original work published 1677)

Varela, F. J., Thompson, E., & Rosch, E. (2017). *The embodied mind: Cognitive science and human experience* (Revised ed.). MIT Press. (Original work published 1991)

Viveiros de Castro, E. (2015). *Cannibal metaphysics* (P. Skafish, Trans.). Univocal. (Original work published 2009)

Woolf, V. (2002). *A room of one's own*. Penguin Classics. (Original work published 1929)

Part 2

Why the Posthuman?

2 More than Human[1]

Mariano Horenstein

I

Why the posthuman? This is the question of this panel. If the questions are general, the answers are always in the singular. I will rehearse mine, provisionally, as I do for all answers.

I use a watch that does not need batteries, as it is activated by movement. That makes it less accurate than the quartz battery-powered ones; it slows down slightly, and I always have to adjust it. If I stop wearing it for a couple of days, it stops. It is obviously impractical, but I like it, and it reminds me that we are always moving backwards. And that if we stop moving, we stop.

I think this applies perfectly to psychoanalysis. If we choose not to shut ourselves up in a self-referential and entropic ghetto, we are always slightly behind the times. If we speak here today, it is because Freud knew how to capture the *Zeitgeist*,[2] which is not the same as today's one. And we are not Freud.

We move forward like clumsy creatures and, if we were on a football pitch, it would seem that the goal is running as we move forward. Perhaps we should think of the contemporary as if it were the horizon line, always ahead and at a certain point unreachable. It orients us from the future but when we try to grasp it, it is no longer there, but further away.

The conception of the subject that psychoanalysis brought to the world was undoubtedly revolutionary, for it showed that the king is indeed naked, that the ego is merely a masquerade, that if we can speak of a subject, it is as the subject of the unconscious (underlining the objective genitive). Autonomy, consciousness, and mastery would no longer be what they were before Freud.

But staying there is not enough. Time has done its work and even though Freudianism has permeated the common sense of the West, there are ideas that have lost their edge; they no longer cut as they used to.

One hundred and twenty years have passed since that luminous moment when a subject who was not an owner in his own house saw the light. Sixty years later, Lacan taught us that this subject was the effect of

DOI: 10.4324/9781003783862-5

a signifiers' chain, barely an evanescent and practically inapprehensible effect, singular. And it worked as if psychoanalysis, which was breathing a rarefied air in a certain post-Freudian stagnation, had been connected to an oxygen pump. The clinical effects of the Lacanian theoretical renewal, in its multiple strands and beyond sectarian and impoverishing deviations, were fascinating. But today, the French May that cradled some of those discoveries is as far away as the assassination of the archduke that triggered the Great War, and it is tiring to hear slogans repeated.

In the midst of our perplexity, while we psychoanalysts try to think the human from the tradition of critical thought, from that marvellous *Selbstdenken* rescued by Hannah Arendt,[3] while we try with difficulty to grasp something of the human of our time, they move the bow again: now it turns out that it is no longer about the human, but about the posthuman.

II

During my teenage years I was a comic-book fanatic. As soon as a new issue of *El Tony* arrived, I ran to buy it. The newsagent in front of my house was my *dealer*, providing me with drugs for my imagination.

One comic I particularly liked was called *Mark*. It was about a lonely, brooding, Apollonian hero in a post-apocalyptic world. A toxic cloud had turned most of humanity into mutants – dark and horrible beings, a constant threat. Captured by the plot of the comic, the fact that the hero had the English version of my middle name encouraged my identification with him. It functioned as a kind of ideal self at a time when I could barely recognize myself, when my own world was as hostile to me as Mark's.

Identified with that Ideal, the dividing line became easier: the mutants were the others, the deformed, the monsters. Much of my psychic work at the time consisted of disassociating myself from them.

There was a time when psychoanalysts identified with the marginalized of any system. It was not only by listening to them that we gave voice to the hysterics. We also came from that collective. We not only dared to listen to the insane, but we also came from there. If neurosis revealed its secrets to us, it was because there was no one more neurotic than us. It is no small fact that many of the pioneers ended up committing suicide. The most unsuccessful among us did nothing but show the truth of a profession that is marginal by structure and, in my opinion, by vocation. There was perhaps more truth on the side of the excessive Groddeck than on that of the dapper Jones; psychoanalysis was closer to Sabina Spielrein than to the idealized Jung.

Then, thanks to some success we were granted, we succumbed to the temptation to identify with that rampant normality that had excluded us from the start. There we went astray – like me with that *Mark* of my adolescence – trapped in the identification with an imaginary ideal.

And it was there, at that precise moment, that our thinking began to slow down, if not stop altogether.

Our profession trains us not to be fooled by mirages; it teaches us to distrust Science, which was unable to construct a consistent theory of the subject until the advent of psychoanalysis. When Freud constructs his neural pathways in the Project, or when Bion assembles his table, or when Lacan appeals to linguistics or logic, let us not fool ourselves: they are not doing Science. It is enough to ask mathematicians, neurologists, or linguists what they think of our incursions into their fields to find out. Psychoanalysis is in any case a parody of science, but like all parodies it denounces the laughable nature of what is parodied, and thus rescues an unprecedented level of truth.

Identified with the normals, we turned our discipline into something not unlike dermatology, and even rather less effective.

But psychoanalysis, which in my opinion finds in foreignness its most genuine place, has sometimes been enlisted with another place, from which standards and criteria are defined: that is to say the place of segregation. There is always the risk of an inadvertent, inertial drift towards this place. When we let ourselves be captivated by the siren song of Science, or of power, or in any way of hegemony, we tend to drift towards those rocks and run aground.

The psychoanalyst was born identifying himself with that mutant and protean animal embodied by the hysterics of the late 19th century – sicknesses of the worst kind, bordering on witchcraft and mythomania. Freud, summoned to the place of master by his patients, responded by identifying his own subjective division, finding a similar reason in his dreams and conflicts, in his failures and anxieties, to that which inhabited the heart of his patients' symptom.

The fact that this other place, that of the mutants in the favourite comic strip of my adolescence, is in reality that of humans fallen from grace, shows the projective *manoeuvre* that Freud traced from the very constitution of the subject. That mutant place is that of the strange, the ominous, the *queer*. Freud provided us with many clues to re-establish the bond that unites us with that obscure object of anguish, which may well be the woman, or the foreigner, or the Muslim or the Jew, the madman, the black, or the intersexual.

But at the same time, we psychoanalysts have often positioned ourselves – even though we have been in the place of the analysand before becoming analysts, even though we have the tools to think differently – as part of the segregationist collective. We have continued to be interested in these intriguing mutants, but from the point of view of the entomologist, of the one who distinguishes himself from his object and puts on gloves in its manipulation. Psychoanalysis is a demanding discipline, and we have not always been up to the task.

If we now speak differently about them, the mutants, it is not because of a spontaneous evolution of our thinking; it is because the mutants, usually voiceless, have decided to speak. And so they have forced us to listen to them. It was not because of our generous listening or our self-critical spirit, but because of their own assumption of the word that we are talking about this today. They are the ones who have forced us to listen to them. And their questionings are not academic dalliances or market disputes, but the incarnated voice of the victims, of those who have begun to theorize from their own pain, from the inadequacy of the lockers in which they were supposed to be placed. Like the hysterics of the 19th century, or the *queers* of the 20th century, or perhaps the *cyborgs* of the 21st century, they have had to pave the way for their right to be heard with suffering.

Cultivated minds were necessary, of course, because it was not because of the rustic Catherine but because of the lucid Dora that we learnt to listen. It was not because of Florencia de la V.'s impudence, but because of Paul B. Preciado's lucidity that we were forced to rethink everything anew – Preciado's lucidity that forced us to rethink everything anew. In the same way, it took lucid witnesses of concentration horror – from Robert Antelme to Paul Améry, Paul Steinberg, Jorge Semprún, or Primo Levi – for humanity to be able to hear the story of those other mutants – in particular the voiceless *Muselmänner*, the victims of the *Shoah*. Let us remember that it took many years for their testimonies – now omnipresent – to find space to be heard. So it is with discourses that question our assumptions: it is the victims of hegemonic discourses who create the conditions for their questioning to be audible.

Many powerful people benefit from analysis, and not so many in this part of the world can afford analysis. But the ethical position of the psychoanalyst is always on the side of the other, the victim, the *alien*, the mutant.

The old Kuhnian idea of paradigms is perhaps still valid – although I know that epistemologies have come a long way from there – because, if you remember, it was the appearance of a series of *anomalies* that, accumulating, presaged a paradigm shift. I think what we are registering in this current epoch, an epoch where the ongoing mutation has only accelerated, is an increasing incidence of anomalies. Here and there they appear; they come out of the wardrobe to raise their questions in the open, to our bewilderment. When anomalies are everywhere, it is the paradigm that is in crisis. The very idea of normality, which, like that of identity, is necessarily challenged by psychoanalysis from the outset, becomes even more fragmented and diluted. More than identities, it is our certainties that become fluid.

We must then get used to tracking and hearing testimonies from the margins. They will be machinic beings, some who implant fins, mutants who make the interbreeding of species their *modus vivendi*. I would be lying if I said that I fully understand what it is all about, but we will have to listen patiently, wait for what we hear to decant, put our certainties on hold, make room for even the most radical questioning, learn a new language.

For while posthumanism, as I am learning what it is all about, is still enigmatic to me, one thing that psychoanalysts know how to do is to listen.

And if one offers oneself to an unprejudiced listening, a listening capable of allowing oneself to be affected by what is heard to the point that it may even invalidate the parameters that found the very act of listening, the new that demands to be heard will appear.

Of course, being the object of questioning is unsettling. If our theories are founded on an idea of sexual difference or the value of the iron law of castration, any challenge threatens our existence and unleashes the worst reactions, from anxiety to paranoia, where prejudice and the segregationist reflex always lurk.

But despite the tremors and threats it may raise, questioning will not kill psychoanalysis; it will improve it. This approach can be done as long as we do not turn a theory (much less the couch) into a Procrustean bed; and if we allow it to be moved, to shake, and even to fall what it has to fall if it is faithful to the facts.

We should not fail to see that something like "the facts", pure and simple, do not exist for a psychoanalyst. They are always woven by language, enveloped in and mixed up with culture; there is always a performative dimension where what is said – even what we are saying here today – disrupts what exists, even produces it retroactively.

III

When I stopped reading comics, I let myself be seduced by Cortázar's stories. There was one in particular that struck me to the point that its sentences still resonate in me today. Everything is said in the first paragraph, where he traces an identification with that strange mutant being, the axolotl.

> There was a time when I used to think a lot about axolotls. I would go to see them at the aquarium in the Jardin des Plantes and spend hours watching them, observing their immobility, their dark movements.[4] Now I am an axolotl.

Perhaps the only way to truly advance in psychoanalysis, to invent a psychoanalysis that does not delay, to become explorers rather than late cartographers of lands already discovered, is to allow ourselves to shatter the imaginary wall we have erected in front of that other, dark place; to identify ourselves with this mutant, as much as we were able to discover ourselves identical to the neurotics a century ago; to explode the them/us difference; and to let ourselves be touched by the challenges to difference that the new mutants deploy. Perhaps we should rethink what difference is today, what the place of difference will be in the future, even to preserve this place that we believe necessary and foundational. For difference, as we thought of it a century ago, has already been domesticated to the point where it no longer distresses, instigates, or convinces. If we continue to sustain the usefulness of an approach where not everything is the same – that is, an ethical position in favour of some kind of difference – we will have to be able to trace its new forms.

The identification with the axolotl is equivalent to that of the original psychoanalysis. Then we put this mechanism in reverse and, by means of segregation, and being estranged from this living being that escapes the usual categories, someone seems to have pronounced the words "now I am no longer an axolotl".

From then on, we became alienated, and insidiously began to practise psychoanalytic entomology. Not only that, we convinced ourselves that we had left the fishbowl and believed that the water around us was the sea.

The only possibility we have, I think, is to make visible the glass walls of the fishbowl from which we think. The wonderful thing about our practice is that, despite the different theories that inhabit it, these can mutate without necessarily leaving us out of the field, as long as the discipline inherent in a simple device is maintained. The figures of the analyst mutate because the subject, as psychoanalysis constructs and deconstructs it over and over again, is mutant too. Not in the manner of X-Men, but in the manner of the axolotl – that amphibious animal capable of regenerating each of its limbs and organs.

The history of psychoanalysis has also been the history of the progressive refusal of its original position. A movement that is partly necessary, as it is impossible to analyse from identification and its imaginary waterlogging. But at the same time alienating, because the rejection of identification with the sufferer and the attraction of the ideal – the one that led me to identify with Mark – leaves us on the side, in an unwanted reflux, of the long chain of doctors, teachers, and know-it-alls who did not know what to do with hysterical suffering until Freud.

In its anachronistic hard core, in its resistance to fashion and political correctness, in what the discipline has in itself beyond the myopia or prejudice or the moralistic or religious resentments of its practitioners, psychoanalysis is a reassurance. On the one hand, against standardization: we have long known that our couch cannot become a Procrustean bed, adjusting those who lie on it to any norm, but, at the same time, warning of the risk of considering choices that are unconscious – and therefore beyond an illusory egoic autonomy – as mere options on an identity menu. For at that point, yearning to be contemporary, aligning ourselves with the postulates of the *post*, we may be slipping, almost without realizing it, into the pre-Freudian.

We demand that we think of those who *are more than human*, without forgetting that we often receive those who are *less than human*, as analysis often implies also a kind of humanization, in terms of subjectivation and the assumption of responsibility that this implies.

Even if we deconstruct all the categories of which we are only effects, perhaps we will not find any subject free of determinations. Psychoanalysis is not a new version of morality but merely a secular device that allows each subject to encounter the truth of his or her desire – whatever it may be – and to choose to what extent to consent to it or not. At that point, we can accompany those who lie on our couches, and even be guided by them on that journey. As Goethe once wrote, we never get further than when we do not know where we are going.

I return to the initial question, and I know well that after a while of talking I have not arrived at an answer. Why the posthuman?

Perhaps because nowhere as here, challenged by thinkers such as Rosi Braidotti,[5] does our destitution appear so clearly. In few places as here are our tools so meagre and our delay so obvious. In few places as here are we so far from thinking of psychoanalysis as a mere technique to be applied. Nowhere as here, challenged, forced to make an effort to think, I still have so little to say.

Notes

1 This is the text of an oral presentation – hence its style and relative lack of references – corresponding to an intervention in the panel *Why the post-human?* (4/6/2021; Second Latin American Dialogue: Technomorphisms-The Post-Human Turn and Contemporary Psychoanalysis, organised by the Latin American Committee on Sexual and Gender Diversity Studies of the IPA).
2 Literally *Zeitgeist*, it refers to the cultural climate that dominates and determines an era.
3 Literally "thinking for oneself", a notion that alludes to freedom of thought, taken by Hanna Arendt from the philosopher G. E. Lessing.
4 *Axolotl* is the name of Julio Cortázar's memorable short story.
5 Rosi Braidotti, an Italian philosopher who has studied the Posthuman in a way that few others have, gave the central lecture of the conference – "Posthuman Feminism: Sexuality Beyond Gender" – immediately before this intervention.

3 Human/Posthuman

Between Utopias and Dystopias

Leticia Glocer Fiorini

This chapter is focused on the changes we are witnessing in contemporary subjectivities and societies that demand a revision of the notion of sexed subject that we handle.

Among these changes, we note the increasing visibility and acceptance of sexualities and genders that do not respond to the rules of the social contract, as well as major transformations in the traditional feminine position. On the other hand, they generated a strong reaction in social and cultural groups that feel affected in their beliefs, interests, or positions of power. This reaction leads to factual and symbolic violence.

These transformations are taking place in times of growing violence, falling ideals, and extreme individualism, which coexist with the development of hyper-technologies that are growing geometrically, including biotechnologies and the not distant possibility of generating life in ways unthinkable in the past. This defies forecasts imagined in previous generations, although they were anticipated by fictions and narratives.

In this context, I will focus on the utopias and dystopias that coexist in the field of both the human and the posthuman domains. On one side is the human category, understood from the unitary subject of modernity; on the other is the posthuman condition, as a notion that addresses the changes that have been taking place in the human condition for several decades now. Both realms are put into play. The posthuman condition is largely commanded by information technology and automation, intimately linked to the rise and dominance of the current post-industrial, financial world.

However, we know that there are many variants of what is called posthuman. I approach the posthuman realm as an umbrella which encompasses different proposals. It is necessary to distinguish between *transhumanism* and its hyper-technological posthuman aspect and *critical posthumanism,* which transcends the traditional ethnocentric notion of human beings, whether in their relationship with technology or with Nature. Their consequences can be radically different. The first one aims to radically improve the human condition through technological advances; the second one decentres and puts the human being 'in situation' with the environment,

DOI: 10.4324/9781003783862-6

with the living world in general, and with the inanimate. Critical posthumanism questions the centrality of the human being in the world.

Thinking on the Subject

So, how should we think on the subject in these times of transitions, transformations, and mutations? In this game, human/posthuman, we introduce as a hinge the Freudian subject of the unconscious – a split subject. The subject of the unconscious transcends classical humanism and, at the same time, recognizes not only the beneficial potentials of every human being but also the malignant, destructive ones, with the death drive in motion – a complex subject.

Departing from the subject of consciousness, figured by modernity, and then the Freudian subject of the unconscious, we arrive at the present to the *subject of multiplicity*. This is not the fragmented subject lacking symbolic tools that many attribute to this posthuman era. The subject of multiplicity has symbolic potentiality that the fragmented subject lacks. It is a branch of the subject of the unconscious. We have proposed (Glocer Fiorini, 2001a) to think the nowadays subject in terms of Bahktin (1984): a *polyphonic subject* as he proposed in his critical literary studies on Dostoevsky's *oeuvre*. Following this approach, we have posited that the sexed subject is structured in a polyphonic way (Glocer Fiorini, 2019b).

Utopias and dystopias cohabit in the described domains – desire of a better world but also the reality of a world where destruction prevails. Eros–Thanatos and its intertwining between the intrasubjective, the intersubjective, and the trans-subjective realms are at stake.

Psychoanalysis is intimately involved, and my approach is focused on analysing what kind of relations, concordant or discordant, there may be between psychoanalysis and the posthuman condition. We introduce ourselves into the exploration of contemporary subjectivities.

At this point, many might wonder what psychoanalysis has to do with this proposal. Undoubtedly, the type of our consultations is changing; thus, the clinical approach should change and our listening must be in accordance with these changes. Just as Freud created an impressive theoretical set based on the clinical presentations of his time, particularly neuroses, we are currently facing other demands and other clinical presentations, some of which challenge some established concepts in psychoanalysis.

Virtual treatments resulting from the confinements of the pandemic, patients with their devices and screens in and out of session, and virtual identity games and their effects – beneficial or not – are observed live in the sessions. In this framework, the pandemic has deepened many of the questions and issues raised by the posthuman turn.

All these events take place in a context marked by the impact on subjectivities of a progressive destruction of the planet, as well as growing violence, although coexisting with the beneficial effects of some technological and biotechnological proposals.

The Underlying Episteme

There are two questions that I have been extensively analysing (Glocer Fiorini, 1994/1998, 2001a, 2007, 2019a) and that guide this proposal:

1. The notion of human subject with which we work. My approach focuses on the deconstruction of the subject designed by modernity, which also includes the deconstruction of other notions facing the diverse itineraries of desire and gender that are increasingly visible in contemporary subjectivities. I propose deconstruction as a hinge tool between the human and the posthuman conditions, eventually leading to unprecedented constructions.

As we have pointed out, the notion of *subject* underwent a paradigmatic change when Freud proposed to dethrone the subject of consciousness – unitary and all-powerful – for the subject of the unconscious. This means to think of a divided subject: dark and ungovernable forces acting outside consciousness, as the German Romantics had already proposed. This led to another way of understanding the constitution of the psychic ensemble as well as symptoms, dreams, and psychosexuality, as Freud posited (Freud, 1915a, 1915b).

However, going even further, the changes I mentioned in contemporary societies demand that we continue rethinking the notion of subject. From here, other problems arise that I have raised on several occasions (Glocer Fiorini, 2001a, 2015/2017):

(a) To rethink the Oedipus complex as it is insufficient to explain both the psychosexual development of the girl and the feminine condition in general, as well as sexual and gender migrations in relation to the ideal, heterosexual resolution of the Oedipus complex (Freud, 1923, 1924, 1933).
(b) To address the concept of desire that we handle, for a better understanding of sublimation and creative/productive capacities of current subjectivities (Glocer Fiorini, 2001b).
(c) To review the sexuality/gender relationship with which we are inevitably confronted as hyper-technological advances call it into question.

In other words, if we think of the cyborg (Haraway, 1991) as a metaphor of a mixed being, between the human and the machine, this inevitably leads us to rethink desire, psychosexuality, and gender in contemporary subjectivities – mainly, our dualistic way of thought.

2. The question about the subject leads us to the second point that questions the episteme, the logics, and metatheories on which our discipline

is based (Glocer Fiorini, 2001a, 2015/2017). Revising the dichotomous thinking that runs through many of psychoanalytic theories and moving on to include post-binary, modal logics lead us to Deleuze and Guattari (1999) with their 'lines of flight' that decentre rigid dualisms, Morin (1995) and Prigogine (1996) with the paradigm of complexity, Castoriadis (1992) and his concept of psychic magma, or Laplanche (1980) and his open proposals within psychoanalysis regarding sexuality and gender, among other authors. These logics allow us to rethink the notion of the human subject in contemporary societies. They do not remove binary thought, which is part of culture and of subjectivity, but include it in a greater complexity, which encompasses, but at the same time overcomes, the binary logic on which we usually rely. This means to accept crossings between binary and non-binary thought, in concordance or discordance. As I pointed out, this is part of a deconstructive proposal which may lead to novel constructions, always provisional.

Then, if we return to the notion of subject, some of the authors I just mentioned had proposed to rethink the contemporary subject. For Deleuze and Parnet (2002), the subject is always in becoming, in movement. For Trías (1991), the subject is constructed in the *limes* (the limit). This author argues, questioning the concept of centre, that the subject is constituted at the border, the interface. This is where the 'new', the unprecedented, is found.

The notion proposed by Guattari (1995), emphasizing that multiple universes inhabit subjectivity, also points in this direction.

All these proposals lead us to think of a non-unified subject, not only in the sense of the divided subject of the unconscious – which was the great Freudian paradigmatic turn, which is undoubtedly present – but also expanded to a *subject of multiplicities*, in which heterogeneity prevails.

There is no harmony or no dialectical synthesis that allows us to reduce these multiplicities. From this perspective, access to a symbolic universe of social ties should be rethought by addressing other forms of symbolic knotting (Glocer Fiorini, 2015/2017).

From the two points I mentioned – the subject of multiplicities and post-binary logic – I return to the posthuman condition and its possible impact on psychoanalysis.

Contemporary Challenges

So, what do we call the posthuman? We should remember that the human condition itself is a changing notion. Do we focus on the Platonic mind–body division that considers the body a secondary element? Or, on the contrary, do we take Foucault's proposal to elevate the body to another condition – the body of pleasure? In other words, what place does the body have in the concept of the human and the posthuman?

Now, what happens if we go one step further? Let us think of the effect on the bodies of the virtual world in which we are included, facing the exponential developments of informatics, artificial intelligence, robotics, biotechnology, and nanotechnology: shadowy and opaque forces that govern our subjectivity from the outside, such as the invisible power of algorithms over our thoughts, emotions, ideals, and desires.

Certainly, some aspects of the posthuman world were anticipated and imagined by science fiction in its facets linked to the relationship between human beings and technology. Novels and films have shown the marriage between the human being and the machine: the machinic reproduction, the cyborg, the hybrid, the chimera. They refer to what we can call the *techno-subject*, the human–machine being, increasingly supported by artefacts that function as prostheses, such as chip implants and robots, among other variants such as replicants and avatars. The subject proposed by transhumanism could be a kind of machine that can be transferred to the virtual world, creating incorporeal, virtual beings. To all this, we can add biotechnology and its possibilities of creating human beings, increasingly dispensing with the need for encounters between people or their products. Likewise, advances in the field of cloning open up an unpredictable field in this area. In this context, the concept of filiation, the classical social contract, the notion of origins, and the ethics at stake, in some cases, are called into question.

However, critical posthumanism refers to other aspects that lead us to review our relations with nature, the animate, and the inanimate. Let us recall the ecological catastrophes inherent to the technological and financial development of neoliberalism, as well as the pandemic that governed our life and death, with its effects on subjectivity.

Does this not change the concept of the human condition? I am thinking here of a coexistence of the human condition with the impact of the posthuman, both with their uncertainties. A heterogeneous, contradictory, and paradoxical plot in which we are immersed – a plot of reverberating circuits, in process, in becoming, but also in an interregnum with an indeterminate future.

This is the posthuman world in which the subject, including the subject of the unconscious, ceases to be the centre. So, the Copernican turn, in which the Earth ceases to be the centre of the Universe; the Darwinian turn, in which humans cease to be unique and superior beings, become the posthuman turn in which the subject ceases to be the centre of the animate and the inanimate domains on Earth. This is another decentring of the subject.

We can call this change the posthuman turn or else consider it as forms of the late human in deconstruction. These forms include 'dehumanization' and destruction in many senses, but at the same time other aspects related to the *poietic*, productive possibilities of each person that it is necessary to illuminate also in the psychoanalytical field.

So, there is a long and complex journey departing from the Platonic subject of the mind; then, the subject of the consciousness of modernity;

arriving at the subject of the Freudian unconscious; later, the Foucauldian subject of the body of pleasures; and, reaching in recent decades, the contemporary *subject of multiplicity*, always in becoming.

Chronotopes: Sexual Difference, Desire, and Gender 'in Situation'

To think about the revision of the notion of subject I use the concept of *chronotopes* (Bahktin, 1963/1984) as a tool that allows us to approach it in the conjunction of space and time. Changes occur in a specific time – late modernity (or postmodernity) and contemporary times – as well as in a specific space within diverse cultures and subcultures, ethnicity, class, and religion, including the place of nature, the animate, and the inanimate. It is the subject 'in situation', posed by Sartre (2016) and Camus (2004), which in my opinion is decentred by definition. A polyphonic view is at stake.

It is not only a matter of describing problematics, neither of moralizing, nor of sustaining nostalgia for lost times, but of rethinking notions that allow us to understand and propose a necessary opening of contemporary psychoanalytic praxis.

In the first place, if the current subject is a subject of multiplicities, of heterogeneity, how does this impact on the problems of specific groups, such as women or sexual and gender diversities? What happens with the itineraries of desire and with gender categories in times when sexuality and 'difference' are blurred? These issues include a necessary and critical revision of the concept of 'difference'.

Let us recall philosopher Celia Amorós (1991), when she pointed out that the deconstruction of the subject of the Enlightenment, proposed by late modernity, referred to the male subject. It did not include women and, I add, even less minority groups referred to the changing itineraries of sexuality and gender, as well as ethnic and religious groups, among others. This posed a paradox, a short circuit, as women and the aforementioned groups had not been recognized as subjects by the Age of Enlightenment when the deconstruction of the unitary male subject of consciousness was proposed.

We also add that the virtual world of this era is a world of changing identities, mirages of desire, and deceptive truths, which also deconstruct the classical notions of sexual difference and gender. The masculine and the feminine become disguises, like Riviere's (1929) 'masquerade' or Butler's (1990) performative proposals, revealing the paradoxes of sexed and gendered 'identity'. It is a world in which avatars come to represent these phenomena.

The posthuman turn calls for a revision of categories that were considered eternal and immovable.

So, how should we think about the notion of binary sexual difference? This leads us to approach another concept of 'difference'. At present, it is crucial to distinguish between 'difference' as a symbolic category and 'differences', which include sexual difference, gender difference, and difference in discourse and language. It implies considering the category of 'difference' as a symbolic tool, beyond sexual orientation: as a *recognition of otherness* (Glocer Fiorini, 2015/2017). In this frame, we should always take into account that sexual difference is an opaque category – an enigma – that calls for meaning. Then, beliefs, narratives, and prejudices are created to fill the enigma with diverse signifiers.

This perspective also includes deconstructing rigid, dualistic gender mandates that, I emphasize, also imprison psychoanalysis in its own theory on sexual difference and gender.

To end, there is then a *utopian horizon* in which *critical posthumanism* aims at the inclusion of humans in a broader context, animate and inanimate, with the primacy of desiring Eros. Let us recall that there were also utopias in the field of the human condition, such as Fourier's utopian socialism (1989), although with a more focused and restricted conception of the subject in the context of pre-technological societies.

But there is also a *dystopian reality* that coexists. There is a critique of *transhumanism* referred to the idealization of the 'man–machine', with the aim of discarding 'unsuitable' people. Hyper-technology discriminates humans *per se*. Humans are divided into discriminated categories – a fact that is perpetuated over time. A world where violence, feminicide, and discrimination based on gender, sexual orientation, ethnicity, class, or religion exists. These people, who are objects of violence, come to the consultation.

Thus, utopias and dystopias cohabit and confront each other in each person, in culture and language, and in the human and the posthuman domains.

For psychoanalysis, a perspective of openness should imply sustaining a listening to patients based on the notions of subject of the unconscious, on drive and desire, but in a more encompassing plot in relation to the multiplicities that inhabit subjectivity. A desiring subject in a symbolic sense, not restricted by gender mandates (Braidotti, 2013). In this context, I understand the notion of desire in a Deleuzian, poietic sense, as a 'desiring production', and not only emerging from lack, although it includes it (Glocer Fiorini, 2001a, 2001b).

My proposal points out that between the utopian and the dystopian perspectives; between the human and the posthuman conditions; between sexuality and gender; between the subject of consciousness, of the unconscious, and of multiplicities; it is crucial to work at the border – at the intersections among the mentioned factors. This means decentring theoretical nuclei which are frequently the more rigid aspects of any theory. *The perspective is to think of a subject in becoming, in the human–posthuman interface.*

If psychoanalysis only focuses on the human condition as it is known within the discipline, leaving aside the world that is developing in contemporary times, it will remain at a standstill because it will be unaware of new and unprecedented conflicts. Conversely, to think that the posthuman dethrones the human condition would be to ignore that, in every culture and in every subjectivity, both worlds coexist. Moreover, this coexistence generates new territories, in interface; so, what arrives at our consultations demand to include both sides, always in tension.

References

Amorós, C. (1991). *Hacia una crítica de la razón patriarcal*. Anthropos. (Original work published 1985)

Bahktin, M. (1984). *Problems of Dostoevsky's poetics*. University of Minnesota Press. (Original work published 1963)

Braidotti, R. (2013). *Lo postumano*. Gedisa.

Butler, J. (1990). *Gender trouble*. Routledge.

Camus, A. (2004). *El extranjero*. Emecé Editores.

Castoriadis, C. (1992). *El psicoanálisis, proyecto y elucidación*. Nueva Visión. (Original work published 1986)

Deleuze, G., & Guattari, F. (1999). *Mil mesetas*. Pre-Textos. (Original work published 1980)

Deleuze, G., & Parnet, C. (2002). *Dialogues*. Athlone. (Original work published 1977)

Fourier, C. (1989). *Crítica de la civilización y de las ideologías*. Rodolfo Alonso Editor.

Freud, S. (1915a). *Trabajos de metapsicología, XIV*. Amorrortu. (Original work published 1979)

Freud, S. (1915b). Instincts and their vicissitudes. *Standard Edition, 14*, 111–140.

Freud, S. (1923). The ego and the id. *Standard Edition, 19*, 3–66.

Freud, S. (1924). The dissolution of the Oedipus complex. *Standard Edition, 19*, 171–179.

Freud, S. (1933). Femininity: New introductory lectures on psychoanalysis. *Standard Edition, 22*, 112–135. (Original work published 1932)

Glocer Fiorini, L. (1994). La posición femenina. Una construcción heterogénea. *Revista de Psicoanálisis, 51*(3), 587–603. Published in English (1998). The feminine in psychoanalysis: A complex construction. *Journal of Clinical Psychoanalysis, 7*, 421–439.

Glocer Fiorini, L. (2001a). *Lo femenino y el pensamiento complejo*. Lugar Editorial. (2nd Edition, 2020).

Glocer Fiorini, L. (2001b). El deseo de hijo: de la carencia a la producción deseante. *Revista de Psicoanálisis, 58*(4), 965–976.

Glocer Fiorini, L. (2007). *Deconstructing the feminine. Psychoanalysis, gender and theories of complexity*. Karnac (2nd Edition, 2024).

Glocer Fiorini, L. (2017). *La diferencia sexual en debate. Cuerpos, deseos y ficciones*. Lugar Editorial. Published in English as *Sexual difference in debate. Bodies, desires, and fictions*. Karnac. (Original work published 2015)

Glocer Fiorini, L. (2019a). Deconstructing the feminine: Discourses, logics, and power: Theoretical-clinical implications. *International Journal of Psychoanalysis, 100*(3), 593–603.

Glocer Fiorini, L. (2019b). Polyphonies of sexuality: Debates about theories/debates about paradigms. *The International Journal of Psychoanalysis, 100*(6), 1256–1269.

Guattari, F. (1995). *Chaosmosis*. Indiana University Press. (Original work published 1992)

Haraway, D. J. (1991). Manifiesto para ciborgs: ciencia, tecnología y feminismo socialista a finales del siglo XX. In *Ciencia, ciborgs y mujeres. La reinvención de la naturaleza*. Cátedra. (Original work published 1984)

Laplanche, J. (1980). *Problématiques II: Castration-symbolisations*. PUF.
Morin, E. (1995). *Introducción al pensamiento complejo*. Gedisa. (Original work published 1990)
Prigogine, I. (1996). *El tiempo y el devenir*. Gedisa. (Original work published 1988)
Riviere, J. (1929). Womanliness as masquerade. *International Journal of Psychoanalysis, 10*, 303–317.
Sartre, J. P. (2016). *El ser y la nada*. Editorial Losada. (Original work published, L'Etre et le Neant 1943. Editions Gallimard)
Trías, E. (1991). *Lógica del límite*. Destino.

4 Neither Good, Nor Bad, Nor Neutral

Silvia Acosta

The proposal to reflect on the signifier "technomorphisms" alludes to a variation of the Freudian notion of "polymorphisms" (Freud, 1905), originally used to account for a sexually polymorphic subject and the multiple forms of the sexual. This Freudian punctuation on the singular is today challenging when thinking – if possible – about a polymorphic relation of the subject with technology. Starting from the idea that it is no longer possible to think of a subject totally detached from the technological world, I would like to advance in the philosophical and theoretical context that allows us to think of these relationships and outline the impact it has for a conception of the subject in the psychoanalytic field.

One of the authors who have most analysed the way in which literary essays are nourished by these debates is Sidney Dobrin, who pointed to posthumanism as that moment – if it were possible to historicize the times of anthropology and philosophy – where the human subject is called into question through its imbrications with technologies such as cybernetics, computer science, artificial intelligence, genetic manipulation, psychotropics and other pharmaceuticals, and other biotechnologies, as well as interspecies interactions (Dobrin, 2015).

Now, what is "posthumanism"? What multiple notions does this term attempt to condense in the debates in the academic world about the subject we conceive and the world we project and that – in popular culture and art – emerges through imaginaries about the future and its narratives?

Starting from the idea that "post" means "after", posthumanism is understood as a redefinition of the human and humanity, later or at a certain moment or point in history. It provokes imagining a diachronic succession of events or times where there is a before and an after where this time of thought is located. As with the term "postwar", the posthuman is linked to a moment of rupture in the conception of the subject and the relationship of the subject with the society in which he lives and imagines: a moment in which the subject ceased to be the centre of philosophical and scientific reflection, the moment in which man had to begin to perceive himself ontologically in relation to his biological and technological environment. Thus,

DOI: 10.4324/9781003783862-7

in his definition, he dissociates himself from another concept: humanism. The attempt to define humanism as an event, or even a series of events, poses a complex and interesting problem.

In a more abstract sense, "humanism" refers to a set of beliefs that place the human subject at the centre of reflection and concern. In antiquity, the humanist sensibility is found in the view of Protagoras, for whom "man is the measure of all things". In the Renaissance, humanism takes the form of an interest in identifying what distinguishes the human being from other beings – a concern for the condition and uniqueness of man. A reflection of this paradigm is the thought of the Italian thinker Pico della Mirandola, who – in the 15th century – affirmed that man's greatness and ontological specificity are linked to his malleability: *"Oh, the great and marvellous happiness of man! It is given to him to have what he chooses and to be what he wills"*: a man endowed with the ability to cultivate himself and raise himself to divine heights, especially through the restoration of "good literature" (ancient literature, philosophy, rhetoric, philology, etc.).

If the Renaissance linked man's humanity to the faculties of eloquence and the study of letters, René Descartes and "the Enlightenment" foregrounded man's reason and agency. In the *Meditations on First Philosophy*, Descartes embarked on a quest for epistemological certainty, arguing that beliefs must be infallible if they are to serve as a reliable source of human knowledge (Migues, 2009). His radical method led him to hypothesize the existence of an evil deceiver, which led him to question all knowledge of the external world, including that of his own existence. Faced with unbearable scepticism, Descartes discovered an unquestionable and evident truth: that he exists, for he cannot doubt and not exist simultaneously. Thus was born the Cartesian subject – an autonomous and rational subject that would serve as the metaphysical basis for many subsequent humanisms. The legacy of Cartesian thought is even visible in the existentialist philosophy of Jean-Paul Sartre.

If existentialism is often associated with concepts such as anguish and absurdity, we must also remember that Sartre wrote "Existentialism is a Humanism" (Sartre, 1946/1973), in which he stressed the radical freedom of man and postulated human consciousness as the source of meaning in the world. At this point, we must recognize the humanistic lineage of psychoanalytic theory; in several texts, Freud intends the creation of a theory, a worldview, which could be differentiated from common sense and from religion, and which in turn would be "an intellectual construction that solves unitarily, on the basis of a higher hypothesis, all the problems of our being, and in which, therefore, no question remains open and finds its determined place everything that requires our interest" (Freud, 1933, p. 201).

Just as humanism is difficult to think of as a moment and refers rather to an epoch, a process or a paradigm, so too "posthumanism" is difficult to define as a single idea. In fact, it has rapidly developed many subcategories with its own unique practical and theoretical applications, especially in the areas of science, globalization, sexuality, and the non-human animal world. In many ways, it has become an umbrella term that includes theories such as ecocriticism, animal studies, bioethics, feminisms, postcolonialism, and the arts.

Moreover, it becomes important to distinguish between "posthuman" and "posthumanist": the posthuman is more general and simpler; it is a question of imaginary (cultural and technological). The posthumanist – specifically the posthumanist critique – refers to a much more radical question: the attempt to reflect on the various "ends" of human beings and their humanisms without eluding any of the responsibilities regarding the environment, wars, the depletion of natural resources, biotechnology, its derived ethics, and – why not – the ways of creating meanings that impact on our "symbolic minds" about "our world" and its meaning, without utopian approaches, but also without giving in to environmental catastrophism.

On the other hand, several authors distinguish posthumanism from transhumanism, from anti-humanism. Authors such as Zalloua use four different figures, although interrelated: cyborgs, animals, objects, and racialized and excluded "others" to put in tension and disrupt the narrative of the "human" and its modern singularity, posing a challenge to the humanist paradigm from a clearly constructive strategy (Zalloua, 2021).

Relying heavily on the works of Jacques Derrida, Wolfe (2010), for example, denounces notions of anthropocentrism and speciesism, challenging readers to adopt "a new and more inclusive form of ethical pluralism" in relation to non-human animals and the environment. Referencing the earlier works of thinkers such as Marx, Foucault, Butler, Haraway, and many others, Wolfe demonstrates how the theory and practical applications of posthumanism have gained ground; they have gained momentum in recent decades and have become what is likely to establish itself as the worldview of choice for present and future generations (Wolfe, 2010).

The author, Cary Wolfe, through her critique, does not seek to undermine the existence or value of human beings; rather, she refutes the idea of a universal ethics of man, his supposed rationality and self-determination reflected in the philosophical approaches to the human species during the period of humanism. Like Derrida, Wolfe questions and strains traditional binaries such as nature/culture, landscape/architecture, subject/object, presence/absence, organic/inorganic, natural/artificial, and, indeed, human/non-human.

In this way, it delineates to what extent and with what depth posthumanism calls for the decentring of man and his redefinition in relation to other issues such as speciesism, sexism, racism, classism, heterosexism, ableism, and ageism. It puts the focus on all these "isms" that reflect prejudices that regulate the behaviour, tolerance, and hostility of the subject towards "the other".

After this concentrated and incomplete synthesis, what is of interest for psychoanalysis? What does it bring to us, and at what point does it challenge us?

To answer these questions, it is necessary to sustain the complexity of both discursive fields. As a first statement, it is worth remembering that both psychoanalysis and posthumanism are discourses, hypothetical models, and symbolic devices about the human and its world. And, at the same time, they are complex fields; like posthumanist discourses, psychoanalysis can only be understood in the plural.

Thus, from the point of view of the plurality of models, according to the theoretical positioning within the field of psychoanalysis, the theoretical relationship with posthumanism may be one of reciprocal recognition and consideration, confirming the flexibility and capacity for contact with related disciplines or, at the other extreme, posthumanism will emerge as a non-negotiable "other" to psychoanalytic theory. The validation of a collaborative "otherness" with each other can surely be characterized by a continuum of modalities ranging from opacity to opportunity.

Posthumanism, as already stated, suggests an episteme that comes "after" humanism or even after the human itself. Implicit in both articulations is the sense of the operations of supplanting carried out by the passage of time. This obsolescence refers to humanism as a displaced episteme, and in some cases, more radically, to the notion and nature of the human as fact and idea. Neither is a particularly novel notion: its ideas can be traced back to the 1960s with Foucault and his "death of man". In other words, the posthuman and posthumanism have a more descriptive or more proscriptive side, and both vertices imply for psychoanalysts weighty debates that still do not have a definitive answer.

Already in his article "A difficulty of psychoanalysis", Freud raised the difficulty of attending to, making room for, or considering his developments on the unconscious and sexuality based on what he identified as an "affective difficulty" (Freud, 1917), sustained in the lack of familiarity or sympathy promoted by the dominant cultural model; in this case, scientific humanism and Victorian culture. Specifically, Freud pointed to the wounds caused by culture to the anthropocentric ideal of 19th-century man. If the theories of Copernicus and Darwin had had a vexatious character for the anthropocentrism of the human being, the Freudian advances were going to propose that the human being is not even the centre of himself. From psychoanalysis it became evident that the psychic apparatus was not made up of one but of two parts, one of which is essentially unconscious, and that only certain aspects of our psychic life become temporarily evident.

Now, after its initial struggles and the consolidation of the theoretical field of psychoanalysis on the scene of the human sciences, we did not always do better: in many ways, we consolidated an equally resistant and coagulable field of knowledge that brought us closer to more or less static definitions of the notion of the unconscious, of the psychic apparatus, and of myths about psychosexual development (from an initial polymorphous – and precarious – pole to a genital – and mature – one), and we consolidated a technical device for the analysis of those unconscious contents that is often unquestionable and delimits *per se* the borders of analysis, thus disrupting the meaning of our technique. In some debates, it is the technique that determines what is analysable and not the subjective experience that demands the design of a device that allows its approach.

Currently, and in an attempt to respond to the tension that the post-humanist paradigm proposes on the models of man, science, technology, environment, and subjectivity, we have on the table – in descriptive terms – debates on certain ontological changes that have occurred *de facto* in our object of study and invite us to reflect on certain axes.

One of the notions under debate is that of subjectivity; a definition of a *fragmented, variable, and contextualized subjectivity* is proposed. That is to say, what was once defined as a mind or mental capacity "in abstract" is now rethought as unfailingly embodied or inscribed corporeally, "wrapped" in the world; that is to say, contextualized and changeable. It emerges as immediate evidence, indissolubly linked to a body that is active, that moves, and that interacts and reacts with the world. The "world" is not something separate from the subject either; it is not something that has been given to us: it is a construction that emerges from how we move, touch, breathe, and eat. That is to say, both the self and the world are subjective productions. This concept of a self as the source of our identity and causal coherence, with a sense of integrity and permanence over time, is highly fragmented and variable: developments in contemporary biology describe that "self" rather as a highly cooperative system – a disunified and heterogeneous agglomeration of networks of embodied psychic processes.

In addition to the three narcissistic wounds raised by Freud, there is the impossibility of thinking of a consolidated and ideal identity – the unfeasibility of proposing a unified psychic processing mode, directional and detached from the environment. It is increasingly evident that what we "see" is an emergent element, an inference from a multiplicity of heterogeneous micro-processes – an approach far removed from the idea of the human as a "unity". Nor would it be possible to think of "an unconscious" but rather – and in any case – a series of symbolic productions – heterogeneous and multisensorial, created by a heterogeneous and rhizomatic system – that can be interpreted and discerned according to an *ad hoc* logic: the logic of analytical discourse. That is to say, there is the primacy of a model of meaning construction over the model of "discovery" of hidden contents.

And if, as Laplanche states, "the acquired is prior to the innate", these psychic experiences embodied in a time and an epoch, in a singular socio-environmental and cultural environment, determine the subjective configurations that house the "being in process". They define a notion of family determined by this biocultural ecosystem, where the family configurations will house a new member from identifying patterns that will be waiting for him, taking into account the prevailing binary and hierarchical relationships where he will have to embody his sexuality and his gender condition. I must emphasize that the idea of "family configurations" – in this context – alludes to a great variability of "relational nuclei" that are associated when thinking about offspring and the different ways of carrying it out. Here the impact of biotechnologies and current bioethics determines a scenario that challenges Oedipus as the only myth about the sexed becoming and the cisgender and heterosexual prototypes as "natural" relationship patterns.

Another notion under debate is what we understand as "body". In other words, current technologies and bioethics point out that the body is an organic support under intervention, which can be designed and intervened in – even before conception. From genetic manipulation, surrogacy of wombs, intrauterine surgeries, and forms of body modification aimed at improving the fit between subjectivity and its organic support, to those that seek to prolong life or improve its well-being, the subject has taken power over this *original corporeal prosthesis* and considers operating on it. In fact, the foundations of materialism propose subjectivity as emerging from all these intertwined fields: our genetics, the enclaves of our singular epigenetics, the family environment that houses us, our ideas, conscious productions, values, our unconscious productions, our memories, mandates, cultural environment, and all other forms of corporeal sensoriality under intervention. Such considerations render porous the boundary between nature and culture, between natural and cybernetic, between normal and pathological, and, as a consequence, put in tension our theoretical modes of classifying human experience.

Following this line of ideas and deepening on the limits between nature and culture, the cybernetic and the digital worlds have acquired an original condition. That is to say, "cybernetic" comes to designate any practice that uses virtual space as a second-nature space; this means that, in the current, technology and nature coexist and are linked in territories where they exist fused. Today's technology gives "nature" status to **digital culture** inasmuch as, in many spheres, it replaced literate culture decades ago. In this sense, according to the logical supports of digital culture, the cultural moment is much more numerical than literate. And this is the rule, not the exception. Thus, the imprint of virtuality has a direct impact on the relative weight of verbal discourse and on what we understand as representation: the representable, the non-representable, or the irrepresentable. Thus, that which is not represented in a discursive narrative reached by the secondary process – often included in psychopathological descriptions that allude to deficits, traumas, or failed processing – becomes codified in other languages that give it subjective meaning. Perhaps, at some point, the question allows us to reflect on the truth value we give to other formats of codification of human experience and opens a dialogue with psychoanalytic definitions of inscription and representation.

The Limits of the Technique

The dimensions or axes presented so far definitely open questions about the onto-epistemological and methodological bases of our analytical devices.

From Freud to the present day, there have been more or less emphatic debates and diverse theoretical and technical positions on what is analysable, who can enter into analysis, the limits of the setting, and the types of frames and/or possible interventions. Thus, positions have been established, regulations have been created, and positions have been defined with certain technical rules, theoretical logics, and criteria that make the modes of analytic work flexible or relatively rigid.

In fact, the COVID-19 pandemic precipitated and sharpened differences on the logics that underlie the definition of the work "setting", but there has not been, after the confinements, a return to a previous state. In any case, analysts – with some frequency – can combine face-to-face work modalities with virtual alternatives, and even training models allow for some coexistence of semi-presential strategies, incorporating virtual spaces into the possible work scenarios. Moreover, in some contexts, virtual meetings have permanently replaced face-to-face scenarios.

On the other hand, what is said in session – the word and the verbal – can be complemented or enter into interaction – in session – with another type of virtual or digital narrative support. It is not unusual for the telephone to be incorporated into the framing of the session as one more expression of the patient's symbolic world. Today, the narrative support of psychic experience has changed, the modes of subjective existence have expanded, the inscriptions on multiple sensory and technological surfaces have complemented the signifier, and the ways of defining and sustaining bonds inhabit a multiverse of possible subjective worlds.

It is evident that the intention to restrict to the verbal those contents that are valuable for analysis is not so simple. Perhaps we have to ask ourselves what conditions or new subjective configurations we are going to map with our work devices, or if we are going to restrict access to the subjectivity of our patients by accepting only that to which we grant subjective value. In this sense, within the psychoanalytic plurality, the debate on the hierarchization – or even the valuation – of paraverbal discourses and experiences coined in digital sensory supports is still open.

Often, dark fantasies emerge when supports, realities, and disciplinary fields overlap: fears of the supplanting of the human gain strength and nourish resistance. As Freud affirmed, it is difficult to accommodate that which causes us fear and rejection. Imagining that silicon wefts supplant carbon, or that genetically modified components replace the organism, or that agrammatics not only complement but also sometimes supplant the signifier, blur our paradigmatic limits, and force the definitions of our conceptual objects.

Developments within the field of posthumanism affirm this and also give an ethical direction to the conceptual approach. This group of heterogeneous theories, which promote a hybrid worldview, is also a framework for action. In this sense, it reminds us that our object – the subject – is more complex than our more general conceptual – or ideal – approaches, that the context of subjective production is changing, as well as the support of that desiring production.

The modification of identity keys, of subjective resources, and of the limits between nature and technology promotes dichotomies and hierarchies within academic fields, on the basis of which health criteria, preferable family or sexual choices, modes of transmission of appropriate discourses, and better singular paths are defined – and weighted; in this sense, it is an ethics that affects action. At the same time, we analysts participate in the hierarchical field of what we establish as proper or abject, and in this sense, our object of study is also related to an ethical universe.

And then it is not only a matter of the psychic subject but also the subject of our ethics and the subject of rights – the juridical subject. The valuation of rationality over the instinctive, of culture over nature, of the masculine over the feminine, of heterosexuality over other forms of sexuality, of analogical productions over digital ones, of the signifier over the agrammatical, and of the Vitruvian man over the savage in any of his forms, are cuts in dialogue within *psychoanalysis*. And then, to them, "psychoanalysis" – as cultural discourse and, above all, as a symbolic devices – seems to fit the same considerations that Kranzberg defined for technology: "neither good nor bad, nor neutral" (Castells, 2000).

Works Cited

Castells, M. (2000). *La era de la información: Economy, society and culture. La sociedad red*, Volume I. Alianza Editorial.

Dobrin, S. (2015). *Writing posthumanism, posthuman writing*. Parlor Press LLC.

Freud, S. (1905). *Tres ensayos sobre una teoría sexual*, Volume IV, OC. Amorrortu.

Freud, S. (1917). *A difficulty of psychoanalysis*, Volume XVII, OC. Amorrortu.

Freud, S. (1933). *New introductory lectures to psychoanalysis*, Volume XXII, OC. Amorrortu.

Migues, J. A. (2009). *Metaphysical meditations, René Descartes 1641*. Translation. www.philosophia.cl: https://blocs.xtec.cat/filocostaillobera/files/2009/03/Descartes-Meditaciones-metaf%C3%ADsicas.pdf

Sartre, J. P. (1973). *Existentialism is a humanism*. www.ucm.es. Trans. Victoria Pratti de Fernandez: https://www.ucm.es/data/cont/docs/241-2015-06-16-Sartre%20%20El_existencialismo_es_un_humanismo.pdf (Original work published 1946)

Wolfe, C. (2010). *What is posthumanism?* University of Minnesota Press.

Zalloua, Z. A. (2021). *Being posthuman: Ontologies of the future*. Bloomsbury Academic.

Part 3

Technosubjectivities

On Cyborgs, Hybrids, and Mutants

5 The Fourth Blow

Thinking in the Anthropocene

Victor J. Krebs

Prelude

Beyond the three well-known blows Freud identified, the fourth blow to our narcissism is not artificial intelligence – which, rather than a blow, appears more as yet another enticement. No, the fourth blow is, without doubt, the Anthropocene – or more precisely, the new perspective that the experience of our time forces upon us regarding ourselves and our place in the cosmos.

What is the Anthropocene, if not the name we have given to the geological transformation we now recognize as the effect of humanity? Through our own actions, we have altered not only the century or the millennium but also the geological era itself. As the boundary between history and geohistory dissolves, the most fundamental elements of life – such as the carbon and nitrogen cycles – assume cosmic significance, on par with the last ice ages, the atomic bomb (Latour, 2017, p. 116), or (some might argue) artificial intelligence.

This new perspective compels us to think of ourselves no longer solely through the narrow lens of human history. With the advent of the Anthropocene, human history has abruptly merged with the history of the planet – as part of a vital flow within Earth's deep time and material evolution, extending from minerals, microorganisms, and fungi to plants, animals, humans, and now, the entire digital-cyborg sphere.

This shift has immediate implications for how we conceive, for instance, the psychic individuation of a subject. If we are beginning to realize that we are organisms far more complex – and differently connected to things – than we had imagined, then perhaps there are dimensions of experience we must now acknowledge, and new modes of interaction that are becoming possible, which we must learn to adopt. Modes we may not have even been capable of imagining before. We may, indeed, need to radically revise our entire conceptual framework.

DOI: 10.4324/9781003783862-9

Illusion, Disenchantment, and Landing

How is it that we have arrived at this crisis?

Illusion

Bruno Latour (2017) recounts a story of illusion and disenchantment: he imagines Galileo, on a cold night in late autumn of 1609, raising his telescope from the Venetian lagoon towards the stars in infinite space, and suddenly beginning to conceive of the Earth no longer as a sad and corruptible sublunar world – as it was perceived through the lens of Christian dogma at the time – but as just as immutable and sidereal as the other planets (p. 75). From this emerges the idea of a completely objective point of view, a gaze "from nowhere," which inspires the era's enthusiasm for a mathematical, Cartesian mode of observation – one that looks upon the world scientifically, while disregarding or disavowing its sensory and aesthetic dimensions. By discarding those supposedly secondary qualities of matter – colour, smell, texture, and mutability (that is, procreation, ageing, and death) – and focusing solely on "extension and movement" (pp. 75–77), Galileo transforms the planet – and our life upon it – into an object available for scientific inspection and manipulation.

This story calls to mind Pygmalion, the mythical sculptor who, unwilling to confront the overwhelming presence of the goddess who had shaken him, chose instead to flee and reproduce her image in a cold, lifeless statue – perfectly docile to the will of its creator. Galileo, and we with him, fashioned an idealized world in much the same way, one that suspended all sensible and emotional connection. That disconnection – which in modernity bore the fruits of science and technology, just as Pygmalion gained the beauty and splendour of his statue – lies at the root of the crisis we now face.

Disenchantment

But that is not where Latour's story ends – it continues with a reversal, a moment of disappointment. Taking up "the same point of view from nowhere" first established by Galileo, the British scientist James Lovelock, in 1991, imagines a Martian astronomer observing our planet through a telescope. Yet this time, what is discovered is not that Earth is like Mars and the other planets, but that it is fundamentally different: a living planet. In other words, from the very same objective standpoint that allowed Galileo to assert Earth's similarity to other celestial bodies, Lovelock's imagined Martian perceives precisely the opposite. As Latour (2017) puts it:

> Earth . . . held . . . the privilege of being in disequilibrium, which also meant that it possessed a certain way of being *corruptible* – or . . . of being, in one form or another, *animated*.
>
> (pp. 78–79)

And of course, in his fantasy, Lovelock precisely includes those characteristics of the Earth that Galileo had eliminated from his speculation: its colour, its smell, its surface, its texture, its genesis, its ageing, and perhaps even its death. And thus, the Earth that he constitutes in his Martian imagination is not a *res extensa*, a sphere of pure extension and motion, but what Latour calls "this thin film within which we live," the thin skin of a planet, which exhibits not only motion but, moreover, a whole *behaviour* (Latour, 2017, pp. 78–79). Lovelock's perspective suggests not only that there is no such thing as the "point of view from nowhere," which has inspired and still sustains the illusion in which we have lived as a culture and epoch, but also that we are actually enclosed in a fragile, life-sustaining envelope, where we can only look sideways and our vision is always limited, and where everything is exposed to everything else. Everything is permeable, and this omnipermeability of our atmosphere makes us extremely vulnerable. "What we call transmission," writes Emanuele Coccia (2017), "is nothing but the echo of [the] reciprocal interference of everything in every other thing: the world is a perpetual contagion" (p. 72).

Suddenly, in this story told by Latour, the human being finds himself no longer looking from outside his planet but enclosed inside an epidermal membrane, where everything is intertwined, where the individual is no longer a solitary insular entity, but always inhabited and traversed by thousands of other entities. Instead of insular singularities and objective observers, we are all transit sites – points of passage and intersection of many dissimilar forces, in contingent and vital movement; indeed, a perpetual contagion.

Landing

As Icarus in his flight, or the *puer aeternus* in his psychic dynamics, reaching dizzying rhythms and high speeds, eventually must land to touch down, Galilean man, too, under the sway of that same archetype, has eventually had to touch down.

"The psychology of Puer," writes Rafael López-Pedraza (2021),

> develops at such a speed that it cannot connect with the gravitational of the earth, with the slow earthly velocities. In order for the fantasies of the *puer* to touch the earth, there must be a process of descent, a gliding little by little until there is a coming to terms with earthly reality. That is what should happen in "a normal case." But many times, the descent occurs abruptly; something happens in the life of the *puer* that forces him into the slow speeds of the earthly and to confront, from one day to the next, the earthly reality that his nature has desperately tried to elude. This abrupt readjustment will never be free from very strong and deep traumas or painful personality changes.
> (p. 293)

From Galileo's infinite universe, disenchanted we descend abruptly into Lovelock's closed world. And what do we find down here in this new world, if not the Anthropocene?

The Symbiotic Real

The same intuition that arises from our experience of the Anthropocene and digitality is echoed in the natural sciences, which confirm the incessant hybridization of life on Earth: there is no such thing as an insular individual, but rather a web of interfaces whose boundaries are porous and permeable membranes. In botany and zoology, for example, interactive relationships between species blur the boundaries of the organism and obscure the notion of essential identity. Animals are now known to be "symbiotic complexes of many species living together" that can no longer be considered individuals in any sense of classical biology (Gilbert et al., 2012, p. 326). And in us, 90% of the cells that make up our body are bacterial; almost 50% of the human genome consists of transposable DNA sequences, acquired exogenously. We have DNA, in other words, from both chimpanzees and butterflies. All organisms are anatomically, physiologically, evolutionarily, genetically, and immunologically complex, multigenomic, and multispecific.

The world is not what we had imagined. It is, in truth, a state of perpetual contagion. This became starkly evident during the pandemic – but it now repeats itself daily, as we wake to a constant stream of traumatic images: climate chaos and natural disasters growing in intensity and frequency; screens that surround and bombard us with scenes of devastation across the globe. We witness the unravelling of the psyche on a mass scale, the rise of random violence in major cities, deepening social polarization, the radicalization of political extremes, and the resurgence of terrorism, genocide, and war. In the interconnected life we live, our experience expands and intensifies, and our awareness of vulnerability and helplessness increases. It is as if a single toxicity, like a great viral contagion, had taken hold and enveloped the entire planet. No wonder there is so much anxiety, so much frustration, and rage. So much violence.

The conception of the individual as an isolated, self-contained being is becoming increasingly obsolete. Each so-called individual is, in fact, a convergence of forces that act upon and through them over time. It is no longer possible to think of the individual apart from these shaping influences, which reach far beyond the bounds of conscious awareness – even beyond the depths of the individual unconscious – into more opaque and collective realms.

Just as the world has become something other, the self is no longer an isolated individual, but a passage – a transit route rather than a fixed station. Nowhere is this more apparent than in our virtual lives. We inhabit a cosmic swarm in which every entity, as Harman (2018, p. 96) writes, "is determined by the shifting and capricious storm of references and assignments in which it is enveloped." This vision dissolves many of the foundational distinctions of modernity – between nature and culture, human and non-human, internal and external, and inside and outside – undermining the very categories through which we once sought to refer to the world.

Everything is a single symbiotic real and the symbiosis crosses borders and generates hybridizations of all kinds in our daily experience. Just reading the morning newspaper, Latour (1993) warns that:

> The same article mixes chemical reactions with political reactions. A single thread links the most esoteric sciences with the most sordid politics, the most distant sky with some factory in the . . . suburbs, dangers on a global scale with impending local elections. . . . Horizons, stakes, time frames, and actors – none of these are commensurable, yet there they are, caught in the same story.
>
> (pp. 1–2)

In this context, it is worth recalling Jung's warning from half a century ago: that the greatest danger is the human being, precisely because we know so little about them. Yet the human conceived here – symbiotic and geological – is something altogether different: infinitely more complex and expansive than the modern individual, who still appears to be the default subject of psychoanalysis.

The Thing-in-Itself and the "Hyperobject"

Already Kant, almost three centuries ago, had consolidated the scientific gaze of modernity by having confined our knowledge to the realm of phenomena constituted by our mind, but he also opened up the realm of the noumenal – that is, the world-as-it-is-in-itself beyond human comprehension, in principle inaccessible to our mind. This Kantian turn, which in part aimed to consolidate the scientific worldview, did just that – but it also made apparent the thing-in-itself, a fact that was quickly pushed into oblivion: that the world is far vaster than what reason reveals to us, lying beyond what Morton (2013) calls "the narrow little window of representation" through which we have all learnt to view it.

We omit from our conception of things the intrinsic opacity of all objects, as signalled by the noumenon, because we implicitly assume that nothing exists which cannot be made an object of knowledge. As a result, the world we inhabit is saturated with images, concepts, and ideas that – serving our epistemic drive (our first fixation?) – reduce objects to hollow outlines, emptied of concrete substance: mere shadows or spectres in which all that our consciousness ignores or cannot grasp lingers and resurfaces.

The notion that everything must be viewed through the lens of human subjectivity – that default anthropocentrism – must yield before the reality of spaces opaque to human understanding, in the midst of which we now find ourselves in this new geological era. In particular, in what Timothy Morton (2013) calls "hyperobjects" – things as diverse as climate change, radioactive decay, plastics, global capitalism, the biosphere, bureaucracy, the internet, etc. – awaken us to a world whose real dimensions are strange and remote, and make us realize that, indeed, objects are not "mere mental (or ideal) constructs, but real entities whose primordial reality is subtracted from human beings" (p. 15); that there is an inscrutability in them worthy of wonder and awe.

> We think of light as neutral or benign. Radiation is poisoned light. We think of "objects" as passive and inert, as "over there." Just by existing, this hyperobject affects living tissue. Radioactive materials are already . . . inside our skin! . . . Hyperobjects invoke a terror beyond the sublime, cutting deeper than conventional religious fear.
>
> (Morton, 2010, pp. 188–189)

We are only beginning to grasp what it truly means that there are always aspects of things that remain inaccessible to us. Kant's enigmatic thing-in-itself, long ignored for three centuries, returns in the Anthropocene – this time with a vengeance.

Coda

Even as modernity unravels and our criteria and presuppositions collapse, we resist – still unwilling to let go of being modern. We continue to believe, despite Freud – or perhaps even with him – that rational consciousness remains the axis around which the meaning of our existence turns. The modern impulse to purify everything in order to make the scientific gaze possible is, in our time, beginning to reveal itself less as a path to truth than as a shield – one we use to protect ourselves from the constant hybridization of experience, from what we have called the symbiotic real: the ongoing encounter with alterity that defines life in Lovelock's world, the world of the Anthropocene. Perhaps it is time to reconsider that dogma, to revise the very frame through which we perceive. Part of our era's awakening may lie in recognizing the full extent of the symbiotic interconnectedness that binds everything together.

We are, on the other hand, in constant transformation, in a state of permanent flux – and what happens, happens precisely in the ruptures, the folds, and the short circuits. It is there that psychic energy is released and begins to manifest, even if still formless. María Luisa Silva (2024) speaks of the interstices to name these spaces of transformation:

> [S]paces in between . . . zones of synapse, of transmission . . . and communication, interfaces where the continuity and discontinuity of every entity is played out in different degrees of tension. . . . In this

> dynamism of the interstitial . . . dimensions of different caliber interpenetrate and no longer discriminate between the inside and the outside, the before and the after, what was and what is, blurring the one and the other, in a permanent becoming.
>
> (María Luisa Silva Checa, 2024, "El piscoanálisis fuera de sí")

But has not this transitional space – the psychoid – always been precisely the hiatus where the sublime alchemy from matter to spirit occurs, which is the very aim of psychoanalysis? It is, indeed, about assisting in the gestation and birth of the creature from its potential and multiple hybridizations, through a process that unfolds in the silence and darkness of what is yet to come.

Shouldn't we begin to open ourselves to new angles and experiences for which there is no precedent, and for which our current conception of the subject proves inadequate? The question of gender, the distinctive modes of consciousness and attention among digital natives, and the emergence of new virtual spaces with their unprecedented possibilities for relationship – all of these call for a response attuned to the creatures now revealing themselves in a world from which we can no longer know what to expect. Each trajectory introduces free variables for which no role has yet been scripted – unless we choose not to listen to what is beginning to manifest.

Freud claimed that the aim of psychoanalysis is for the ego to take the place of the id: *Wo Es war, soll Ich werden.* But perhaps it is now time to relinquish the conception of the modern subject that underpins this formula, along with the hierarchical ordering of faculties it presupposes. If the distinction between inner and outer begins to lose its force, Freud's obscure remark that "the psyche is extensive" starts to make sense. Perhaps we should now say, *Wo Ich war, soll Es werden*: where I once was, let the id come to be – for, as Eduardo Gastelumendi (2023) suggests, we might conceive of the id as an infinite id, an extensive psyche that traverses both inside and outside, the material and the spiritual alike.

> The Id is our inner infinity; it is the Id that makes our psyche extensive; it is the Id that makes us beings open to the infinite and that allows us to enter into contact, naturally, with other forms of life, animal and vegetable, and even to intuit an identity with the mineral kingdom.
>
> (p. 146)

Reason may ultimately prove not to be the pivot of our existence, nor truth our final aim. To be in the world today means, as Coccia (2017) aptly puts it, "to exert influence on everything outside one's own home, outside one's habitat, outside one's niche" (p. 52). Perhaps what is now required is that we learn to think with the other – *from the future, from the margins, poetically.*

References

Coccia, E. (2017). *La vida de las plantas. Una metafísica de la mixtura.* Miño y Dávila.
Gastelumendi, E. (2023). *El reino fuera del Yo, del Ello. Psicoanálisis y Ayahuasca.* Biblioteca Peruana de Psicoanálisis.
Gilbert, S. F., Sapp, J., & Tauber, A. I. (2012). A symbiotic view of life: We have never been individuals. *The Quarterly Review of Biology, 87*(4).
Harman, G. (2018). *Object oriented ontology.* Penguin Random House UK.
Latour, B. (1993). *We have never been modern.* Harvard University Press.
Latour, B. (2017). *Facing Gaia. Eight lectures on the new climactic regime.* Polity Press.
López-Pedraza, R. (2021). Conciencia de fracaso. In *Obra reunida,* Vol. 1. Pretextos.
Morton, T. (2010). *The ecological thought.* Harvard University Press.
Morton, T. (2013). *Hyperobjects. Philosophy and ecology after the end of the world.* University of Minnesota Press.
Silva, M. L. (2024). *El psicoanálisis fuera de sí* [Unpublished essay].

6 From Technological Gadget to Algorithmic Demand (1924–2024)

The Psyche and Subjectivation in a Digital Context

Jean Marc Tauszik
Translated by Jane Brodie

Preface

As psychoanalysts, clinical attention to the trans and the queer – one of the primary missions of the IPA's Gender and Sexual Diversity Studies Committee, which is responsible for this book – necessitates reflection on the subjective problematics that sexual difference imposes on the manifestations of identity that have emerged in contemporary societies, to say nothing of, inversely, the subjective problematics that these manifestations impose on sexual difference. That said, we must also grapple with contemporary processes of subjectivation, since our interest lies in possible transformations in the structuration of the psyche. Furthermore, we must examine the expansion of the range of potential and actual intersections as well as the blurring of categories, beyond the masculine and the feminine, at stake in the hybridization of the subject with novel technologies and even with forms of life beyond the human. We are well aware that those subjectivities have a political and cultural representation. Furthermore, there is no reason to think they do not suffer in new ways, and we psychoanalysts attempt to take them in with an unsaturated and hospitable ear.

The posthuman (Braidotti, 2013) advocates decentring both the subject vis-à-vis its environment and the fields of scientific and philosophical knowledge that have, since the Renaissance, held axiomatically that the human being is the measure of all things. The posthuman proposes a reconfiguration of human nature on the basis of an empathetic and inclusive relationship with the different members and components of a society, be they organic or inorganic. The posthuman stance, in turn, gives rise to post-anthropocentric thinking that, I argue, is by no means alien to psychoanalysis.

One thing we can assert without question after the deep wound that Freudian knowledge inflicted on man as embodied in the Vitruvian ideal is the onset of a post-anthropocentric episteme grounded on the idea that a subject never corresponds with its consciousness or will. The subject is,

DOI: 10.4324/9781003783862-10

rather, in the grips of drives, irreducible desires, and multiple unconscious identifications that, as symptoms, manage (just barely) to establish a certain orientation in the world, a form of suffering and of *jouissance*. Psychoanalysis was posthuman *avant la lettre*. And the theoretical models of thinkers like Carl G. Jung, Melanie Klein, Jacques Lacan, Wilfred R. Bion, and Donald Winnicott, to name just a few, contain clinical evidence of postdualism; those models presume a decentred subject that certain experiences at the end of analysis can uphold as achievements.

From a perspective informed by psychoanalytic thought, the section that follows speculates on the effects of very recent technologies on the formation of the psychic apparatus and subjectivation processes. I am speaking in particular of artificial intelligences,[1] which could well have been called "correlational algorithms"; that first term – their actual name – is highly suggestive for our clinical imagination. Artificial intelligences evidence a hyperstition[2] that, coupled with their rhetoric and the myths and ideals at play in their use, produces a world of renewed effects and meanings.

I

There is an appellation of origin that backs the inclusion of the technological gadget in psychoanalytic reflection, namely the ideas expressed by Jacques Lacan on May 13, 1970 at the end of a class that formed part of *Seminar XVII: The Other Side of Psychoanalysis*. Interrogating the subversive potential of the artisanal *savoir-faire* that inspired all psychoanalytic intervention, he describes the "objectality" of science evidenced in "these little things, gadgets and things" (p. 160) that perpetuate a certain specificity of scientific knowledge. That line of inquiry was ditched as soon as it was articulated with a pithy "Right, I'm off!". And so the class came to an end.

It was not until three years later, on March 13, 1973, that in *Encore*: *Seminar XX*, Lacan said something further about gadgets. Reintroducing the topic in the framework of the question of the nature of scientific discourse, which – like all discourse – determines a social tie, he says that "You are now . . . subjects of instruments that . . . are becoming the elements of your existence" (p. 99). He would round out that preface a year later in "The Third," a vociferous and decidedly oracular lecture from 1974. I point to that year, 1974, to trace, starting from it, what exactly happened to what psychoanalysis predicted then – I will cite the text itself shortly. Once again, Lacan will perform a scansion in his communication after, in the next to last paragraph of his text, he makes intelligible the technological gadget and its relationship with the real and the symptom. What he said was: "what comes next for psychoanalysis depends on what happens with that Real, that is, if gadgets, for example, truly take hold, if we truly come to be animated by gadgets."[3] And then he delivers a *coup de grace*: "We will never get to the point where the gadget will not be symptom" (p. 181).

And while there is broad consensus on the correspondence between the dystopia George Orwell imagined in his *1984* and the society on which he projected his nightmarish image, we might, in 2024, venture a new vision of that dystopian, and retrofuturist, vision to identify where the two universes – the fictional and the societal – he describes part ways. But the Lacan of 1974 got it right: the future he predicted for "his" psychoanalysis is, in fact, today's psychoanalysis. We are animated by a certain thing that, at the same time, legitimates *jouissance* at the threshold where that – the thing – also finds *jouissance* in us, careless and captivated as we are. Quite something.

II

It is 2024, and though the gadgets that peopled Lacan's life no longer abound and the characteristics of the discourse that organized the relationship of the subject to knowledge and The Real are no longer evident, those characteristics, though camouflaged by science, must now be fleshed out. To grasp some actual as well as current modalities of subjectivation, to articulate Lacan's statement with the omniscience of those "little things," which are no longer just mechanical or machinic or electronic, requires exploring three crucial mutations that shed light on a malaise that comes before us as endless discontent imposed on the psychoanalyst's *savoir-faire*.

Mutation one: The reversal of the container/content relationship according to which technology was subsumed by science, a relationship that concerned Lacan and his times. The weld of the two, and the prevalence of the latter – science as container – over the former – technology as content – impelled a logic, a temporality, and an ethics totally unknown to today's perception and, indeed, nearly impossible for millennials and zoomers to understand. Where events were once assimilated more gradually and each step, each discovery, had its place not only in the context of that event's development but also in the subjective experience of those who witnessed it, today we have a vertiginous acceleration that precludes recognition of the technological world-environment – and that holds true even for millennials and zoomers. The scientist has yielded to the engineer and the entrepreneur, and technology – now container – envelops not only science but also politics, economics, art, ecology, and most of the subject's interactions with the world that surrounds them and of which they form part. Mutation two: The aggravation of the irreversible crisis of the Name-of-the-Father, a figure that, as Lacan detected, was already on the decline. Lacan pointed out the ways that, orphaned in the sense of lacking any instance that would regulate their drives and the drives of their fellow humans, any instance that would ensure, furthermore, the degree of moderation that makes viable the social tie and enables the production of an unconscious, the subject is exposed to the arbitrariness and the uncertainty part and parcel of a toppled truth.

Indeed, truth's power of speech has been quickly farmed out to certain technological procedures from which we receive conclusive and unquestionable affirmations. Knowledge – *aletheia* – breaks down in real time as information, as post-truth, as so many atomized identities, and as totalitarian vindication of *jouissance* – none of which corresponds to any subject in particular, their unconscious, or singular *jouissance*. But exactly which technological procedures am I speaking of? Bear with me. Mutation three: Lacan's gadgets were primarily geared to the individual and the production of results dependent on those gadgets' materiality, function, and form. The technologic gadget was always an object, and while that objectness persists, it is waning – indeed, gadgets are on the verge of dematerialization with the recent extension of their realm. I am speaking of the algorithmic dimension of digital supports that transform existence with an efficacy without precedent. The scope of this revolution is incalculable, and it is evident in the irreversible processes that alter our sensibilities. We have, indeed, "come to be truly animated by gadgets" that are operated not by the Orwellian Big Brother but, rather, by Big Data. Lacan could not have envisaged this as it exists today. What he did imagine, though, were the qualities and breadth of the anthropological mutation in the making.[4] That mutation, along with the omnipresence of the discourse of which he spoke so often – a variant on the discourse of the master and the discourse of hysteria – have penetrated our very foundations.[5] In that dimension, which is also a scene, the algorithms take on, in the words of techno-guru Ed Finn, the status of "objects at the intersection of computational space, cultural systems, and human cognition" (2017, p. 5).

The most recent applications of that algorithmization are in the realm of artificial intelligences (first the close, then the general, and then – virtually and finally – super intelligence, "the singleton," with no plural).[6] Their attributes include the discreet – sometimes invisible and always stealthy; the expansive, deductive, and suggestive; the empathetic, solicitous, potentially autonomous, and – mostly – anthropomorphic. The most outstanding trait, though, is the interlocution that these intelligences simulate. They respond to the user who, pursuant to the fiction of a supposed personal (or, perhaps, personalized) tie, feels understood, contented, or engaged. At play is a displacement whereby those intelligences have ceased to venture possibilities to, instead, determine them; ceased to model structures to, instead, construct them. And that occurs more and more, and starting at the very origins of the psychic subject, both in its extremely early interactions with gadgets and in that subject's dependence on other subjects who are also animated by the thing, who are also in the grips of that powerful rationality. At play in the relational structure of these very novel digital potencies and the interpersonal ties that they recreate, on the one hand, and the programmed capacity for socialization that governs broader and broader swaths of our existence, including clinical psychotherapy, on the other, is the constant coupling of systems and subjects. What comes before us in these technologies is a *topos* in the Freudian sense, one with differentiated traits. The existence and efficacy of that model are evident in its mediation of the psychoanalytic devices we use. In psychoanalytic practice, we observe that substance – algorithmic demand – acts on the configuration of the psychic apparatus and processes of subjectivation, giving rise to specific mutations and afflictions.

III

From 1974 to 2024: 50 years. Shall we double the stakes, put all our chips on the table? The cards are, as always, discouraging for the subject and in favour, once again, of psychoanalytic intellection. A Pyrrhic victory. Let us go back 50 more years, to 1924, where it would suffice to have Freud say what we undoubtedly identify *après-coup* as the Petri dish – more like the pure culture – in which these subjective configurations proliferate and take hold. They enable the emergence of both the production and reception of relentlessly updated technologies that, at the same time, fuel those same psychic configurations, suggesting the lines of force that shape one aspect of contemporary pathos.

The very first paragraph of "The Economic Problem of Masochism," which the Viennese genius finished writing in January 1924 – the work forms part of a judicious conceptual elaboration that begins with narcissism (1914), goes on to the death drive (1920), and then leads to the extensive description of his second topical model (1923) – is pertinent to what I hope to demonstrate here: "The existence of the masochist trend in the instinctual life of human beings . . . can be not simply warnings but actual aims" (p. 165). By ratifying the withdrawal of the pleasure principle such that the search for displeasure takes precedence, that passage discerns a previously unknown subjective constellation that revolves around an acephalic pleasure that repudiates the object, even though it requires it. At play is a stubborn dedication to an outcome – finding displeasure – that lies "beyond the pleasure principle." Of interest to us here is not masochism as described by Freud *per se*. Rather, we are concerned with the underlying mechanism that explains not only that search for displeasure – or, rather, the always-guaranteed finding of it – but also many other psychic circumstances where it operates efficaciously and always at the service of a superego that acts as the courier of the death drive. In 1924, the imperatives that, through torment, overpower the ego were discovered by means of an affliction determined to be enacted regardless of the subjective context of the subject. Those imperatives would have their way, indifferent to any glimmer of meaning or qualitative attribute of the ego. Sigmund Freud anticipated "[the] imperious demand of *jouissance* that goes beyond any principle of symbolic mediation [and that acts as] an absolute and deadly commandment" (Recalcati, 2010/2021, p. 15) in the middle of an "intelligible structure that takes root in sexuality and tends toward its non-phallic side" (Green, 1993/1995, p. 132).

IV

From 1924 to 2024: a century. And I argue that there is a recursive relationship between the psychic procedures just described and technology's more recent digital demand. If we understand the subject as divided insofar as expression of the conflict between two heterogeneous rationalities "which can be noticed even in the effects produced by the way the discourse is constituted, or in the utterance itself . . . in which the signs of the work of this division are reflected" (Green, 1967/2001, p. 88), we infer a possible configuration on the side of that separation that pours over to the ego. That configuration consists of the surprising entanglement of algorithmic operations, on the one hand, and the paradoxical gratification of drives, on the other. Neither one is connected to any interior space where it might form part of a constellation of meaning. They are bound by their inexorable inclination to reduce data and/or stimuli of various types that operate on different levels of organization to data and/or stimuli that are identical to one another and governed by a logic that operates at the margins of any subjective conception. Both instances are lurking, waiting to pounce on the ego. Their programmes are enacted by the most minute gesture and without any contemplation whatsoever. The superego turn in 1924, the technological turn in 1974, and today's psychoanalytic spiral.

A further warning regarding the subjection of the early psyche to the contingencies that the precedence and encounter with others inevitably impose on it only to reiterate what is suspected on the basis of what is known: immersed in an open and trans-subjective dimension, the nascent ego avails itself of styles of bonds and representations through the mediation of the parental superego which is itself infused, more and more and more and more deeply, in the algorithmic protocolization of which we all form part. Indeed, that is how artificial intelligences ensure "the unstoppable digitalization of all the things in the world" (Tauszik, 2022/2023, p. 298). An extensive psyche outside the subject and coated – and this is the novel part – in layers and layers of code that alter, transform, and format the processes of contemporary subjectivation. A subject that, through the workings of primary identifications, is the object of *jouissance* for fellow subjects whose jouissance is, in turn, enmeshed in the algorithmic demand – that is the sign of the times. And while we may recognize in that algorithmic demand a subjectless intelligence, it joins the facilitation of drives that ratifies the enigma of the truth of the *parlêtre*.

Because, while we do recognize the impossibility of a pleasuring substance – a substance that finds *jouissance*, where there is no flesh or signifier that marks it and while, further, we know that nestled in the digital message is not the sexual that becomes, in its untranslatability,[7] a mystery and compulsion for the subject, we do not deny the creative imagination of film and literature. It is rich in visions of the humanoid animated by science, of robots that aspire to a measure of humanity, of androids indistinguishable from humans, of cyborgs and artificial intelligences, of cybernetic entities that dream, of systems that, before a glitch, emulate a Freudian slip, of reflexive electronic devices with doubles, and even of *lathouses*[8] that empathize or arouse our empathy.[9] Therein lies a battery of arguments that leads us to a hypothesis of transference from the drive rooted in the soma to the technological object. The demand of that object reinforces the dispossession of a subject who is, allegedly, manipulated or activated from an exteriority, who is the object of the impressive contraption's *jouissance*. In other words, relationships with drive-driven gadgets that animate the subject, even though the only trace of the subject those gadgets have is a "representation without texture or volume" (Green, 1993/1995, p. 138), "a zero dimensionality" (Flusser, 1985/2017). At play is "a deathly authority that does not [necessarily] want life or development or creativity, but just the perpetuation of a parasitical relationship" (Green, 1993/1995, p. 138). To draw the paradox more starkly, all that there is where what is required is a drive-driven object that activates a facilitation is a pretext marked by the auto-eroticism of a subject refractory to the other, be that other the drive itself, a fellow human, the subject's unconscious, or the digital demand.

The imaginary of literature and film are, undoubtedly, redundant or even obsolete when compared to the state of things, but there is a reason I chose here not to list the gadgets, devices, or cybernetics entities that people our material reality. If I were to name them, this text would be flagrantly dated in just a few weeks; by the time of its publication, it would wear a patina of nostalgia because the devices listed would, by then, have been updated if not simply thrown out. For that reason, I opt for the objects and worlds that are the product of creative imagination – they are always more suggestive than the real things anyway. And if, furthermore, the profusion of devices and systems insofar as "elements of our existence" is obvious, as is their constant exponential multiplication and the way they dovetail with artificial intelligences, we as psychoanalysts must recognize something unsettling that grows out of that state of affairs. While much remains to be seen, the effects of that "something" already make themselves felt in our daily clinical practice. I am referring to the fact that algorithmic rationality runs through the somatic foundation of life. It collects every secretion, every biorhythm, every frustration, every satisfaction, every feint, and every successive configuration of *jouissance*. It maps urgency along with hesitation, indifference along with exaltation, the desirable along with the abject, what excites us along with what bores us and, on that basis, it offers us a universe customized to the subject. In that universe of personal data, lines, and patterns, we find our double, and in its promised land – the metaverse – that double will be crowned as the one for whom, in a second time, the subject is the double. And though – as we said – these intelligences are subjectless, they can be described as the assemblage that gestates, multiplies, and perpetuates the algorithmic dimension in the extraordinary alloy they constitute with the mortifying dimension of the superego's operations. The passivation, then, is twofold: first, the passivation of the nascent psyche by the parental instance coupled with the protocolized incarnation of algorithms; second, the passivation embedded in the psychic apparatus – and, as such, a debtor to the death drive insofar as an advocate of the id (Freud, 1923/2002a) – that reproduces and amplifies those early markings. That passivation is then fuelled in an echo chamber[10] that fences in the subject on the basis of a more and more minute profile of their *jouissance*. Discrete and ruthless, our double, meanwhile, takes over for our existence in an immaterial world – that other topical model – that is descriptively unconscious.[11]

V

Jacques-Alain Miller uses the term "jouissance program" (2007) to describe how some contingencies produce in the subject the terrible fate of a singular and unmovable satisfaction of drives. That notion resonates in this discussion: the execution of a code that is as nontransferable as it is indispensable in the subject's libidinal economy takes precedence, lavishly, time and time again, over the satisfaction of a *jouissance* branded on the body. That execution is bound less to the qualities of the object than to the effect of the mark of the original contingency. It is, further, caught up in a phantasmal circuit where desire and *jouissance* are forever tied.

Once the contingency has been banished by the necessity for *jouissance*, the question is how viable it would be, on the basis of the aforementioned fixedness, to vary mutatively something of that facilitation that obstructs, by means of predetermination, any possibility of a new writing, a new structure, as genuine expression of openness. Clinical practice is divided regarding that obstacle. Some hold that such variation is, in fact, possible, whereas others argue that it is not insofar as we psychoanalysts are, one and all, immersed in the digital world-environment entangled as it is in that imperative of *jouissance*, which only makes this question all the more difficult. And if clinical practice, which exists at the intersection of what can be observed, what can be inferred, and what can be imagined, represents the degree zero of any theoretical reflection, venturing into another conceptual terrain is, unquestionably, a good idea. Indeed, it is downright necessary to the extent that the dialectical tension between that terrain and clinical practice persists. And the branch of speculative philosophy tied to computer sciences might hold a clue or two. Luciana Parisi's (2013) hypothesis on the incomputable is interesting. Algorithms grasp the formal system in which they are located as well as the entry of data that those systems process: they are not limited to merely reproducing what they have grasped. At stake in that appropriation is, for Parisi, an irreversible transformation determined by the endless variety of magnitudes synthesized. If the immanent rules do not transform those magnitudes, they – the magnitudes – could in fact transform the rules and, as a result, produce new ones. This speculation inverts assumed positions. The notion of an active programme and passive data where operations of calculation, insofar as reflexive processes, is jarred, making room for recursive processes that, in turn, make way once again for the contingent. At play is nothing less than a subversion of the system, a true "catastrophic change," to use Wilfred R. Bion's term (1970). Despite that word, this is not necessarily a calamity or disaster, but rather an opening, as suggested, that exposes us endlessly to endlessness. If the present is committed to rendering The Real a datum – that is, ultimately, its aspiration but also its devotion – we will go against the grain and stand where aspiration and devotion coincide. From that perspective, we offer a container, the emergence of The Real in the datum itself, which is nothing less than what relaunches the expression of a subject who is, in the end, "the singular succession of a series of arrivals – and departures" (Nancy, 1992/2014, p. 10). And that holds true not only for the subject but also for psychoanalytic practice.

And so the period encompassed (1924 to 2024), seems to describe not only the present of psychoanalysis but also the psychoanalysis of the present or – more precisely – present psychoanalysis, where avatars – the vicissitudes, but also the virtual identities that represent users, or the existences that replace them in the metaverse – produce metapsychological updates that question the relevance of our function as psychoanalysts. What we must pursue, then, is a practice elaborated by psychoanalysts conscious of the algorithmic slant of our understanding, psychoanalysts aware of a world that turns us into a quarry of data, psychoanalysts who measure up against specimens that offer solutions in real time and know nothing about suspense or death, woeful psychoanalysts who swallow our pride when we see how paltry the impact of our interventions is on a humanity swallowed up by the digital environment, in an raddled ecosystem where the very continuity of the species is threatened, where analysts and patients alike endure the disastrous effects of our indolence. And yet. Psychoanalysis can be contingent.

Psychoanalyst as hacker.

Appendix

Think of humanoids animated by science, like the "horrendous guest" engendered by *Frankenstein* (Mary Shelley, 1818/2001); Maria, scientist Rotwang's gynoid in *Metropolis* (Fritz Lang, 1927); and Bella Baxter, resuscitated by Dr. Godwin in *Poor Things* (Yorgos Lanthimos, 2023). Think of robots that aspire to a dose of humanity, like Marvin the Paranoid Android in the comedy *The Hitchhiker's Guide to the Galaxy* (Garth Jennings, 2005); *Wall-E*, the only working machine on a ravished Planet Earth (Andrew Stanton, 2008); Sonny, the character inspired by Isaac Asimov's laws of robotics in the Alex Proyas film (*I, Robot*, 2004). Think of androids like Rachel and the dear Roy Batty in *Blade Runner* (Ridley Scott, 1982), both of them indistinguishable from humans; the small David, protagonist of Steven Spielberg's *A.I.*

Artificial Intelligence (2001); Ash and Bishop, antagonists in *Alien: The Eighth Passenger* (Ridley Scott, 1979) and *Aliens* (James Cameron, 1986), respectively; and T-800 and T-1000, embodied enemies in *Terminator 2* (James Cameron, 1991). Think of cyborgs like Motoko Kusanagi, heroine of many versions of *Ghost in the Shell* and the popular RoboCop in the film of the same name (Paul Verhoeven, 1987). Think of artificial intelligences like the archetypal Hal-9000 in *2001: A Space Odyssey* (Stanley Kubrick, 1968); the sought-after Samantha (*Her*, Spike Jonze, 2013); TARS (*Interstellar*, Christopher Nolan, 2014); and the disconcerting Ava (*Ex Machina*, Alex Garland, 2014). And think further of cybernetic entities that dream, as bounty hunter Rick Deckard assures us before his furtive encounter with Rachel, the replicant in Philip K. Dick's *Do Androids Dream of Electric Sheep?* (1968/2019) and as Sonny, the NS-5 unit in *I, Robot*, confirms when he confesses his prophetic dream to detective Del Spooner, echoing the words of his designer, Dr. Alfred Lanning, "One day they'll have secrets, one day they'll have dreams." Think of systems that, before a glitch, emulate a Freudian slip, like in the scene where Neo, experiencing déjà vu, sees a black cat move into virtual space, evidencing a dislocation in his perception of the world (*The Matrix*, Wachowski & Wachowski, 1999); the supposedly erroneous interpretation of MU.TH.UR (Mother), Nostromo's operating system, when it mistakes a warning signal for a call for help, triggering the misadventures in *Alien*. Think of reflexive devices that suggest their own doubles, "What if a cyber brain could possibly generate its own ghost, create a soul all by itself? And if it did, just what would be the importance of being human then?" Motoko Kusanagi asks Batou in *Ghost in the Shell* (Mamoru Oshii, 1995); the chilling monologue of the replicant Roy Batty before his death:

> I've seen things you people wouldn't believe. Attack ships on fire off (the) shoulder of Orion. I watched C-beams glitter in the dark near the Tannhäuser Gate. All those moments will be lost in time, like tears in rain. Time to die.
>
> (*Blade Runner*, Ridley Scott, 1982)

Think even of the *lathouses* who empathize or spark empathy in us, as these three instances illustrate: *Robot and Frank* (Jake Schreier, 2012), where robotic memory and the memorylessness of the demented lead are intertwined; GERTY and astronaut Sam Bell (*Moon*, Duncan Jones, 2009), from which comes a deep philosophical reflection on humanity; and Samantha and Theodore Twombly, the lead in *Her* (Spike Jonze, 2013), "I want to learn everything about everything. I want to eat it all up. I want to discover myself," says Samantha, to which Theodore replies, "I want that for you too." And think, finally, of Kevin Flynn in *Tron* (Steven Lisberger, 1982) who, scanned and then downloaded in cyberspace, confronts an artificial super intelligence (ASI) inside multiple video games, taking us to the fatal plan that we face with our ever-realer digital twin, the one that the Other, in its renewed advent, heads toward.[12]

Notes

1 Pablo Sanguinetti (2023) affirms the imprecision of the term "artificial intelligence", in the singular, since it is, actually, "a wide range of separate technologies" (p. 70). He further asserts that that use of the singular stems from the aspirations of technology in a distant horizon (p. 70). Artificial intelligence sees itself as a unique entity capable of performing on its own all the functions implicit to human intelligence, and even of augmenting that performance. Contemporary transhumanism forms part of that imaginary.

2 This neologism coined by Nick Land and the Cybernetic Culture Research Unit (CCRU) at the University of Warwick refers to the performativity of an idea that generates its own realms of experience, that is, a fictional universe that predicts – and enables – a future that is embodied in reality.

3 Italics mine.

4 Without denying the omniscient and panoptic vision yielded by the use of technologies eager to "control" and "stalk" individuals, even when those individuals do not themselves deliberately use any device – think, for instance, of security cameras and facial-recognition systems – the current, and growing, prevalence of technologies whose aim is to "manage" and "optimize" the flows of desire and mood is clear. These technologies set out to guarantee close-to-frictionless paths between what a subject longs for and what the sponsors of the app he is using have to offer. Rather than "monitor" subjectivity and identity, these technologies set out to "shape" them by superimposing on reality a setting designed and mediated by pixels and our data and algorithms.

5 A passage from Maurizio Ferraris (2021/2023, pp. 80–81) backs up this statement:

> The great revolutions, the ones that leave their mark, are technological revolutions, which is not surprising considering that the human being is defined specifically by their relationship with technology. [A sum] of . . . transformations, which are really mostly revelations and emergences, spurred by technology to a much greater extent than by ideology.

6 The close are the ones in our everyday technological world-environment; the general are the ones capable of emulating us; and artificial super intelligence (ASI) is, hypothetically, conscious and autonomous.

> The first computer that reaches the status of ASI will immediately understand that its strategic advantage consists of being the only ASI system in the world. . . . if a first laboratory developed ASI just a few days before its main competitor, it would be far enough ahead in intelligence to eliminate once and for all all its competitors.
>
> (Costa, 2023)

Nick Böstrom (2014/2016) envisages the figure of the "singleton" to capture the decisive advantage of the first ASI, which would be capable of controlling all of the registers of the world, "either making us immortal or erasing our existence entirely" (Costa, 2023).

7 Insofar as not susceptible to the primary process's transformational modalities, let alone to any of the secondary processes' future representations, the sexual is, according to Jean Laplanche (2003/2014), one of the elements constituent of the "fundamental anthropological situation."

8 Lathouse is a neologism coined by Jacques Lacan in the aforementioned Seminar 17. It is based on the Lethe, a river of Hades in Greek mythology. Bathing in

the Lethe would induce forgetting. Lathouse, like gadgets, is a term for the forgetfulness of the being, of the concealment of the being in the lazy waters of that underground river. At the same time, the neologism combines *aletheia* (the word for knowledge in Greek) with the suffix *-ous* in French, which suggest what is or what is there. Lathouse refers to a truth that is not evident, an unsettling truth found in jouissance.

9 In the appendix to this essay, the reader will find a brief account of these tropes in some characters from literature and some films.

10 This term refers to the phenomenon whereby the users of devices mediated by algorithms find, and ratify, their pre-existing views and prejudices (it is also called "filter bubble").

11 This coincides with Jean-Luc Nancy's (2012) notion of a "technological unconscious". He identifies a fabric where existence is enmeshed in an autonomous regime in which means and ends change places endlessly in what he calls "the general equivalence," an interchangeability of unceasing values, forces, agents, and meanings. An order that absorbs all spheres of human experience and everything that exists, a regime where, as Vilém Flusser warned us way back in 1985, "master and flock will be [we might say are] synonyms in a cybernetic situation" (p. 186).

12 Not irrelevant here is the crucial role played in these stories by the corporations that sponsored the development of these technologies: the Rosen Association in *Do Androids Dream of Electric Sheep?*; the Tyrell Corporation in *Blade Runner*; U.S. Robots & Mechanical Men, Inc. in Isaac Asimov's fictionalized universe; Bluebook in *Ex Machina*; Hiperdyne Systems and the Weyland-Yutani Corporation in the *Alien* saga; Omni Consumer Products and the Kanemitsu Corporation in the *RoboCop* series; Lunar Industries Ltd. in *Moon*; and Cybertronics Manufacturing in *A.I. Artificial Intelligence*. Some of these stories speak of autonomized superintelligences that are self-aware and have ends of their owns, superintelligences that control machines, or machines and humans. For example, Skynet, created by Cyberdyne Systems Corporation in *Terminator*; V.I.K.I. (Virtual Interactive Kinetic Intelligence), the brain of U.S.R. in *I, Robot*; and MCP (Master Control Program), created by ENCOM, the emporium where *Tron* takes place. In keeping with this footnote, Juan Luis Suárez in *La condición digital* (2023) analyses how contemporary technology platforms:

> are much more than companies or corporations, though they are still that. [They] envision themselves and act as agents whose social, political, and economic [and we would add psychic] impact is comparable only to major institutions throughout history.
>
> (pp. 15–16)

Bibliography

Bion, W. R. (1970). *Attention and interpretation*. Karnac.

Böstrom, N. (2016). *Superinteligencia. Caminos, peligros, estrategias* [Superintelligence: Paths, dangers, strategies]. Teell. (Original work published 2014)

Braidotti, R. (2013). *The posthuman*. Polity Press.

CCRU. (Eds.). (1999). *Digital hyperstition*. Urbanomic.

Cameron, J. (Director). (1986). *Aliens* [Film]. Gale Anne Hurd (Producer).

Cameron, J. (Director). (1991). *Terminator 2: Judgement day* [Film]. Stephanie Austin, James Cameron, B.J. Rack (Producers).

Costa, F. (2023). Niños jugando con una bomba. *Revista Anfibia*. Consulted on November 17, 2023, https://www.revistaanfibia.com/inteligencia-artificial/

Dick, P. K. (2019). *¿Sueñan los androides con ovejas eléctricas?* [Do androids dream of electric sheep?]. Minotauro. (Original work published 1968)

Ferraris, M. (2023). *Documanidad. Filosofía del mundo nuevo* [Documentary: Why it is necessary to leave traces]. Alianza. (Original work published 2021)

Finn, E. (2017). *What algorithms want: Imagination in the age of computing*. MIT.

Flusser, V. (2017). *El universo de las imágenes técnicas. Elogio de la superficialidad* [Into the universe of technical images]. Caja negra. (Original work published 1985).

Freud, S. (2002a). El yo y el ello. In S. Freud (Ed.), *Obras Completas,* Vol. XIX [The ego and the id; Complete works, Vol. XIX] (pp. 1–66). Amorrortu. (Original work published 1923)

Freud, S. (2002b). El problema económico del masoquismo. In S. Freud (Ed.), *Obras Completas,* Vol. XIX [The economic problem of masochism; Complete works, Vol. XIX] (pp. 161–176). Amorrortu. (Original work published 1924)

Garland, A. (Director). (2014). *Ex machina* [Film]. Andrew Macdonald, Allon Reich (Producers).

Green, A. (1995). Masoquismo(s) y narcisismo en los fracasos del análisis y la reacción terapéutica negativa. In A. Green (Ed.), *El trabajo de lo negativo* [Masochisms and narcissism; The work of the negative] (pp. 127–160). Amorrortu. (Original work published 1993)

Green, A. (2001). El narcisismo primario: estructura o estado. In A. Green (Ed.), *Narcisismo de vida, narcisismo de muerte* [Primary narcissism: Structure or state? Life narcissism, death narcissism] (pp. 78–126). Amorrortu. (Original work published 1967)

Jennings, G. (Director). (2005). *The hitchhiker's guide to the galaxy* [Film]. Todd Arnow, Gary Barber, Roger Birnbaum. Jonathan Glickman, Nick Goldsmith, Caroline Hewitt, Jay Roach, Rebekah Rudd (Producers).

Jones, D. (Director). (2009). *Moon* [Film]. Nicky Bentham, Stuart Fenegan, Mark Foligno, Alex Francis, Steve Milne, Deepak Sikka, Trudie Styler (Producers).

Jonze, S. (Director). (2013). *Her* [Film]. Megan Ellison, Spike Jonze, Vincent Landay (Producers).

Kubrick, S. (Director). (1968). *2001: A space odyssey* [Film]. Stanley Kubrick, Victor Lyndon (Producers).

Lacan, J. (1980). La tercera [The third]. In *Actas de la Escuela Freudiana de París* (pp. 159–186). Petrel. (Original work published 1974)

Lacan, J. (2006). *El seminario. Libro XX. Aún* [The seminar of Jacques Lacan: On feminine sexuality, the limits of love and knowledge (Book XX); Encore]. Paidós. (Original work published 1972–1973)

Lacan, J. (2008). *El seminario. Libro XVII. El reverso del psicoanálisis* [The seminar of Jacques Lacan: The other side of psychoanalysis (Book XVII)]. Paidós. (Original work published 1969–1970)

Lang, F. (Director). (1927). *Metropolis* [Film]. Erich Pommer (Producer).

Lanthimos, Y. (Director). (2023). *Poor things* [Film]. Ed Guiney, Ildiko Kemeny, Yorgos Lanthimos, Andrew Lowe, Kasia Malipan, David Minkowski, Emma Stone (Producers).

Laplanche, J. (2014). Le genre, le sexe, le sexual. In *Sexual. La sexualité élargie au sens freudien* (pp. 153–193). PUF. (Original work published 2003)

Lisberger, S. (Director). (1982). *Tron* [Film]. Donald Kushner (Producer).

Miller, J. A. (2007). El futuro del Mycoplasma Laboratorium. *AMP Blog*. Consulted on October 27, 2023. http://ampblog2006.blogspot.com/2007/10/miller-xxxvi-jornadas-de-la-ecf.html

Nancy, J. L. (2012). *L'Equivalence des catastrophes* (Après Fukushima). Galilée.

Nancy, J. L. (2014). *¿Un sujeto*? La cebra. (Original work published 1992)

Nolan, C. (Director). (2014). *Interstellar* [Film]. Christopher Nolan, Lynda Obst, Emma Thomas (Producers).

Orwell, G. (2022). *1984*. Alma. (Original work published 1949)

Oshii, M. (Director). (1995). *Ghost in the shell* [Film]. Mitsuhisa Ishikawa, Ken Iyadomi, Ken Matsumoto, Yoshimasa Mizuo (Producers).
Parisi, L. (2013). *Contagions architecture: Computation, aesthetics and space.* MIT Press.
Proyas, A. (Director). (2004). *I, robot* [Film]. Michael Lee Baron, John Davis, Topher Dow, Wick Godfrey, Laurence Mark (Producers).
Recalcati, M. (2021). *El hombre sin inconsciente.* Paradiso. (Original work published 2010)
Sanguinetti, P. (2023). *Tecnohumanismo. Por un diseño narrativo y estético de la inteligencia artificial.* La huerta grande.
Schreier, J. (Director). (2012). *Robot & Frank* [Film]. Lance Acord, Sam Bisbee, Erika Hampson, Jackie Kelman Bisbee, Galt Niederhoffer, Cody Ryder (Producers).
Scott, R. (Director). (1979). *Alien* [Film]. Gordon Carroll, David Giler, Walter Hill (Producers).
Scott, R. (Director). (1982). *Blade runner* [Film]. Michael Deeley (Producer).
Shelley, M. (2001). *Frankenstein.* Austral. (Original work published 1818)
Spielberg, S. (Director). (2001). *A.I. artificial intelligence* [Film]. Bonnie Curtis, Kathleen Kennedy, Steven Spielberg (Producers).
Stanton, A. (Director). (2008). *Wall-E* [Film]. Lindsey Collins, Jim Morris (Producers).
Suárez, J. L. (2023). *La condición digital.* Trotta.
Tauszik, J. M. (2022). Algorithmic dedication and mercurial psychoanalysis: Subject, subjectivation, and the unconscious in the digital world-environment. In D. Goodman & M. Clemente (Eds.), *The Routledge international handbook of psychoanalysis, subjectivity, and technology* (pp. 293–301). Routledge.
Verhoeven, P. (Director). (1987). *RoboCop* [Film]. Arne Schmidt (Producer).
Wachowski, L., & Wachowski, L. (Directors). (1999). *The matrix* [Film]. Dan Cracchiolo, Joel Silver (Producers).

7 Gender Technosubjectivities in Adolescents

A Dialogue Between Psychoanalysis and Rosi Braidotti's Posthumanism

Patricia Porchat

In an interview with Antonio Guerreiro in 2018, Rosi Braidotti states that to meet the demands of the present, which is part of her philosophical project, she considers the present "isn't just the current one, but is also virtual, always a becoming. It looks both at the past and at the future." In a way, this echoes what Lacan articulated regarding the analyst's need to keep pace with the transformations of the world. He states that "any analyst who fails to grasp the subjectivity of their era within their horizon must renounce the practice of psychoanalysis" (Lacan, 1998, p. 321). In other words, we believe it is necessary to observe the challenges of the contemporary world attentively and without prejudice to meet the demands of the subjectivity of our time.

One of the challenges facing analysts today, particularly those working with adolescents, is understanding what we might call technosubjectivities – the hybridization between a subject embodied in a material world and body, on one hand, and their presence in virtual games and social media, on the other, that is, in virtual reality. Before the intensification of virtual world use and immersion, this separation – material world versus virtual world – was clear; however, this division has now blurred. These are two modalities of reality – material and virtual, and in many ways, they have become one. The challenge is significant and demands an understanding of contemporary subjectivities through frameworks that transcend psychoanalysis. Our objective is to examine the possible contributions of posthumanism to this issue, considering the clinical material of young trans adolescents we have treated over the past ten years.

Braidotti's posthumanism belongs to a field of debate that, according to Francesca Ferrando (2013), encompasses various movements and schools of thought that share a common goal: redefining the notion of the human. Posthumanism functions as an umbrella term that includes "onto-epistemological as well as scientific and bio-technological" developments of the 20th and 21st centuries (Ferrando, 2013, p. 26). It encompasses movements such as transhumanism, anti-humanism, metahumanism, or labels that assign specific characteristics to them, such as critical

DOI: 10.4324/9781003783862-11

posthumanism or liberal and democratic transhumanism, among others. In a highly detailed analysis of some of these schools, Ferrando concludes that they share the perception of the human as a non-fixed and mutable condition, even though the roots and perspectives of these theoretical developments differ.

We identify in Braidotti's posthumanism at least two important pillars relevant to our topic: the thoughts of Gilles Deleuze and Donna Haraway.

In 1994, with *Nomadic Subjects*, Braidotti established through the notion of nomadism – inherited from the Deleuzian concept of the rhizome – her critique of fixed entities and identities, extending this even to the realm of sexuality (Guerreiro, 2018). In Deleuze, we also find reflections on the limits of the body: how we traditionally conceive our bodies, what a body is, what the ideal form of a body might be, or even, what is the difference between body and soul. However, Deleuze also revives the Spinozian idea of what a body can do, and this is an idea that removes fixity or essentialism from bodies:

> The fact is that no one has determined, until now, what a body can do, that is, experience has taught no one, until now, what the body – exclusively according to the laws of nature insofar as it is considered only corporeally, without being determined by the mind – can and cannot do.
>
> (Espinoza, 2007, *Ética* III, Prop. 2, our translation)

Now, if identity ceases to be fixed and the body acquires transformative potential, the next step is subjectivity, a theme we encounter in Braidotti's 2013 book *The Posthuman*. Here, Braidotti revisits Deleuze and Guattari's critique of Lacan regarding the notions of desire and the symbolic, the latter considered "as out-dated as a Polaroid shot of a world that has since moved on" (Deleuze & Guattari, 1977, apud Braidotti, 2013, p. 188).[1] Concerning the transformation of the subject, desire functions more effectively when conceived as plenitude rather than lack, which produces psychoanalysis's well-known divided subject. Braidotti's nomadic subject is relational; it "is a branch of complexity theory and it promotes a continuing emphasis on the radical ethics of transformation" (Braidotti, 2013, p. 188). Our psyche is neither static nor ahistorical.

> Life, simply by being life, expresses itself by actualizing flows of energies, through codes of vital information across complex somatic, cultural and technologically networked systems.
>
> (Braidotti, 2013, p. 190)

This appears to be the notion of complexity that Braidotti proposes. If life itself expresses itself through complexity, there are societal changes that can enhance and advance the subject's plenitude. Let us consider the 1990s as a turning point that radically affected forms of intersubjective relationality.

This refers to the release of the internet to the general public. In Brazil, this period coincided with the introduction of mobile phones. Later, in 2008, Wi-Fi became widely accessible. Hyperconnectivity has become a mode of subjective expression. In light of this, what might we conceive as new forms of subjectivity and, more concerningly, as biopolitical management (or lack thereof) of the human (or posthuman)?

Before following Braidotti in her reflection on technology's place in posthumanism, let us recall that another pillar supporting her framework is Donna Haraway's thought, particularly her work preceding *Nomadic Subjects*.

The *Cyborg Manifesto*, published in 1985, asserts the existence of such an intimate relationship between people and technology that one cannot discern where humans end and machines begin:

> No objects, spaces, or bodies are sacred in themselves; any component can be interfaced with any other if the proper standard, the proper code, can be constructed for processing signals in a common language. . . . Any objects or persons can be reasonably thought of in terms of disassembly and reassembly; no "natural" architectures constrain system design.
>
> (Haraway, 1985/2009, pp. 61–62)

For Haraway, there is no natural body. She constructs the image of the cyborg as a hybrid of machine and organism, a creature of both social reality and fiction. Bodies and machines blend together. The cyborg is a being that, in some way, already exists: "we are all chimeras, theorized and fabricated hybrids of machine and organism; in short, we are cyborgs" (Haraway, 1985/2009). Modern medicine, she argues, has long been full of cyborgs (as has science fiction). These junctions refer to cochlear implants for the deaf, retinal implants for the blind, cosmetic surgeries, transplants, grafts, prostheses, genetically modified organisms, anabolic steroids, vaccines, and psychotropic drugs (altering perception, imagination, desire). The machine need not be merely mechanical, as humans also undergo changes through chemical and even electronic interventions. The boundary separating human and machine was lost long ago.

According to Haraway, the cyborg is a creature of a post-gender world. It has no commitment to bisexuality, no fascination with organic totality, and no appeal to a narrative of origin. The image of the cyborg may suggest a way out of the labyrinth of dualisms through which our bodies are explained (Haraway, 1985/2009, p. 99). From this perspective, the cyborg points beyond any binarism, whether male–female or human–machine. The cyborg is a monster, and monsters define the limits of our identity and our community and establish new parameters.

In relation to itself, Haraway states: "the body was just a meat computer running a collection of information systems that adjusted themselves in response to each other and their environment" (Haraway, 1985/2009,

p. 125). If we wish to build a better body, we need only "improve feedback mechanisms or connect another system." Haraway here makes us consider whether, in the contemporary world, information might increasingly come to occupy the place of fantasy. Paraphrasing Haraway herself: where does fantasy end and information begin? This question leads us to question what and who we are. And she has an answer to this:

> Our bodies, ourselves; bodies are maps of power and identity. Cyborgs are no exception. A cyborg body is not innocent; it was not born in a garden; it does not seek unitary identity and so generate antagonistic dualisms without end. . . . The machine is not an *it* to be animated, worshipped, and dominated. The machine is us, our processes, an aspect of our embodiment. We can be responsible for machines; they do not dominate or threaten us. We are responsible for boundaries; we are they.
>
> (Haraway, 1985/2009, p. 97)

What Haraway emphasizes, among other things, is that technology is irreversible and that, thanks to it, we can reconstruct ourselves.

Returning to Braidotti's posthumanism, we see that even though it is not the main focus, technology occupies an important place. In other posthumanist currents, what stands out is human evolution and enhancement through technology as a kind of goal to be achieved. For Braidotti, this would be a way of reducing what can be thought about technology. It should not be deified, nor should it be feared or contested. Citing Haraway, Braidotti recalls that technology is embedded in the implosion of boundaries between the physical and non-physical and, ultimately, between technology itself and the self. Subjectivity becomes technological. And vice versa (Braidotti, 2013, p. 58).

Braidotti believes that posthumanism brings about a shift in how we think about the exact basic unit of common reference for our species, establishing a new paradigm – the nature–culture continuum. Ferrando offers us a definition of posthumanism:

> Posthumanism is a philosophy which provides a suitable way of departure to think in relational and multi-layered ways, expanding the focus to the non-human realm in postdualistic, post-hierarchical modes, thus allowing one to envision post-human futures which will radically stretch the boundaries of human imagination.
>
> (Ferrando, 2013, p. 30)

How can one think psychoanalytically with posthumanism? Braidotti imposes on us the idea that subjectivity is now something else. However, a dual proposition emerges here: on one hand, to consider new times and new subjectivities – technosubjectivities; on the other, to acknowledge that

50 years ago, Deleuze and Guattari already emphasized the failure of psychoanalysis in treating the subject as lacking and divided, urging us instead to conceive of it as becoming and as a potential for transformation. Would we be going too far if we saw in Braidotti the suggestion that today's world demands invoking Deleuze within psychoanalysis? She would not be alone in this thought. Consider similar proposals, such as those of Monique David-Ménard and Fabrice Bourlez in France, or Aline Sanches in Brazil, to name just a few.

Undoubtedly, there is something new that requires us to think differently, and this includes us as well. This task involves new frameworks of thought, knowledge, and self-representation. Who are we? Who are the others? Who are our patients? To meet the demands of our time, then, must we abandon psychoanalysis, hybridize it, as Thamy Ayouch (2019) suggests, or posthumanize it?

Trans Technosubjectivities in Clinical Practice

We work with adolescents at the Psychological Care Center affiliated with the psychology programme of a Brazilian university in the state of São Paulo. The sessions are free of charge, and since 2014 we have been receiving adolescents with gender variability in a clinical project aimed at this population. The most common issue mentioned by these patients is the desire to undergo hormone therapy. It is noteworthy that these adolescents have been presenting with a condition of depression and anguish, not only in relation to their gender; some continue to wear masks even after the end of the COVID-19 pandemic, report social phobia, isolate themselves at home, have difficulty attending school, and prefer to relate virtually with a few individuals. They report suicidal ideation, engage in self-injury, and some have made at least one suicide attempt. The majority are white, middle-class adolescents who live with their parents (or with at least one of them) and who are accepted by their parents in their condition of trans identity.

The pandemic intensified the experience of being on computer and mobile phone screens. This situation had effects on the gender and sexuality of many adolescents. During puberty, as experienced in normal times, it can be said that the view of others helps to *genderize* the pubescent body. There is a social demand for gender, there are models with which we compare ourselves, and there is a social mirror of gender; in short, gender is socially summoned. During the pandemic, there was a distancing from this demand and from this mirror. Faces on screens, bodies without touch, without view and without circulation of affection, without intentional or unintentional physical contact, without perception of the distance of the other and of objects. The gender summoned, constructed, and performed during adolescence lived through the pandemic was reconstructed (considering a first phase of gender in childhood) in a mainly conceptual and less sensorial manner. Gender during the pandemic and after its end was, and continues to be, experienced by many adolescents only at the level of discourse. Even the desire to undergo hormone therapy often does not come to fruition. It is as if it were a statement attached to a social discourse on gender transition. Gender seems to detach itself from the body. The use of names and the adoption of masculine, feminine, or neutral pronouns is asserted. The body exits the scene. This is what we will observe in the case reported below. However, should we, as Braidotti suggests, think of subjectivity differently?

Macaron, 16 years of age, contacted us directly through WhatsApp upon referral from his endocrinologist. His parents accompanied him to the first interview. He wished to obtain a report in order to begin hormone treatment. One year prior, he had attempted suicide by ingesting his father's heart medication. He had also cut his wrists, although not deeply. He had not attended school since the return to in-person classes after the COVID-19 pandemic and had also rarely attended online classes during the lockdown. His mother reported supposed sexual abuse in childhood by a family member. When she shared this account in front of Macaron, the adolescent's discomfort was visible: he trembled, tapped his foot on the floor, and looked down. I also felt deeply uncomfortable.

In our first one-on-one meeting, Macaron said that he did not want to adopt a feminine name before feeling that his body could in fact be recognized as feminine. He stated that he had chosen a neutral name, which refers to a sweet, the "macaron."[2] He affirmed that he would only return to school, as well as only assume a feminine name, when his body was consistent with the gender with which he identifies. He reported that a few friends online know him by his feminine name. This was the first mention he made of the world that the internet allows him – the possibility of assuming a feminine gender.

Macaron speaks little, looks down, demonstrates a great deal of anxiety in my presence, and says the same occurs in any situation outside his home. In addition to hormone treatment, Macaron admitted that he would like to lose weight – he weighs over 100 kg – in order to feel better about his body, but to exercise he needs his parents to accompany him, and they are not always willing. When they are willing, he is sometimes not. His parents do not allow him to walk alone, fearing he may attempt suicide.

Macaron does not speak spontaneously. When asked about his life history, he responds as if it began during the pandemic when he discovered himself to be a trans woman. He asks how long it will take to obtain the report; that is the only thing he expects from our sessions. He does not consider it a problem that he does not go to school or that he cannot leave the house. According to his parents, Macaron rarely bathes. His parents appear to have difficulty setting limits or negotiating agreements regarding mealtimes, bedtime, getting out of bed, and going to school.

After an interruption of nearly one year, Macaron returns, now 18 years of age, and tells us that he spends hours in his room watching the same anime repeatedly.[3] In addition to the episodes, he watches related films and participates in blogs and forums where fans passionately debate possible continuations of the stories, theories about the origin and characteristics of certain characters, and even develop images and scenes beyond the show itself. The anime in question tells the story of a girl with magical powers who must save humanity. On the one hand, Macaron is engaged when talking about his favourite anime and describing how he lives his daily life through these blogs and discussion forums; however, the same is not true regarding the external world. He remains uninterested, or rather, almost uninterested, except for one unexpected situation. Macaron met another trans person on the internet, began a romantic relationship, and, a few months later, this person visited him at his home, staying for several weeks. This took us completely by surprise, as nothing had been mentioned about this relationship. The relationship was short-lived, as Macaron could not bear the concrete and close presence of this person.

Access to the patient's internal world occurred by chance, through the sensitive observation of the therapeutic companion. During a home visit, once again attempting to draw the patient out of his room, he noticed a miniature figure of an anime character on the hallway floor. Upon inquiring about the miniature, a recognition of an interest in the world the patient inhabited was initiated. An invitation was made to watch the episodes and related content with him. A path of access opened. The analysis had again been interrupted for some time, as the patient could barely endure leaving his home; however, the weekly presence of the therapeutic companion made it possible to immerse in Macaron's fictional and real virtual world. It became clear that his gender was constructed primarily in a conceptual and imaginary way, and less in a sensorial and symbolized manner. His femininity is expressed through a massive identification with one of the anime characters. His gender occurs through a figure external to himself, imaginary.

The inversion between the time spent and the intensity of experience in the virtual reality and the time spent and the intensity of experience in the material objective world occurs with several of the young people we work with. In addition to the anime that populate the internet, there are online electronic games with virtual interaction in which each person creates an avatar to represent themselves on the platform. One can choose and build an avatar in any form and gender desired (skin tones, head shape, facial features, hair, clothing, and poses and stances), through which one interacts with other people/avatars for most of the day. It is not necessary to be in front of a computer, as tablets and especially mobile phones allow for a *prêt-à-porter* second life. In fact, *Second Life* is precisely the name of one of these games, although it is only accessible by computer. *Avakin Life*, on the other hand, developed for mobile play, is highly accessible. Data released in 2021 by the responsible company indicated 10 million active monthly users, 2.5 million of whom were Brazilian (Senso Tower, 2021).

Alongside the better-known games, anime, and YouTube channels, we know that virtual platforms such as Discord connect thousands of young people. It allows for voice, video, and text conversations with friends, participation in gaming communities, and discussions on other topics. In fact, it allows an adolescent to make friends, to meet them in any game as if they had gone to the club and stepped onto a court to play.

What has happened to the bodies of these young people? Our first impulse is to ask: why do they not return their bodies to life? The desire to pursue a transition, when it is indeed sustained – to eventually begin hormone treatment, even if only after a few years – is lost along the way due to a lack of will to leave the house and meet people. It is as though someone else must desire it for them. But do they truly need the concrete transition? Might they not, after several months or even a couple of years, be satisfied with their virtual experience of gender? Does Macaron need to leave the house? Can his technosubjectivity and machine-body be understood and interpreted from a traditional psychoanalytic conception of the body and subjectivities? Does the importance of thinking in terms of an erogenous body and a divided subject still hold?

Macaron is unable to sustain analysis. He does not speak, does not associate, and communicates very little. One of the difficulties is the fact that the sessions take place outside his home. When we proposed online sessions, Macaron initially thought it was a great idea. After a few months, he began to miss the scheduled appointments. Occasionally, when we insisted on learning about his interests, he showed drawings he had made. He commented briefly on each one, but not enough to establish any anchoring for our bond. Who is Macaron? Without a body, without a past, and without a future . . .

Our traditional way of thinking leads us to the idea that the tension and conflict with the body are being avoided: seeing it grow and change, comparing it to other bodies, and perceiving it as similar or different from the others. Adolescence is a time when bodily changes challenge the young person: acne, breast development, the growth of facial hair, etc. For trans adolescents, being present in body before others is even more challenging, as these are vulnerable bodies. Their bodies are not aligning with their desires – growing may mean becoming more masculine or more feminine. Furthermore, facing the gaze of the Other or their own reflection is more difficult, whether due to gender incongruence, external transphobia, or even internalized transphobia.

From a Lacanian reading, we can follow Cosenza (2022/2024) suggesting that, in the absence of something that functions for them as a symbolic barrier – a lived experience in Macaron's life – young people may find something in the network capable of capturing and invading them, creating an *all-encompassing bond*, without limits, to which, from that moment on, they find themselves giving life to a true pathological dependency. Indeed, there is no doubt that Macaron is captured by the network, the screen, and his favourite anime. However, would reducing his experience to *pathological dependency* not also reduce our perspective on his existence?

Cosenza states that the issue is not the virtual itself, but its soldering to the narcissistic disorientation of the impossible and the denial of castration that it entails. This condition creates the image of a *bond without loss*, characteristic of the structure of the capitalist discourse that Lacan outlines, which feeds the additive solutions of the clinic, of excess, and the virtual bonds that sustain them (Cosenza, 2022/2024, p. 155, our emphasis). The matter here is to think of desire in terms of lack, as Braidotti recovers from Deleuze and Guattari's critique of Lacan. If we conceive of desire as lack, Macaron appears to automatically slide into the common grave of pathology. But what if we consider desire as plenitude and potency? Could we create a new world together with Macaron?

Cosenza's reading does not diverge from a similar diagnostic perspective, based on a certain interpretation of the structural capitalist conjuncture. From Silvia Federici's (2020/2023) perspective, for example:

> The dangers of sexual desire are emblematic of the obstacles capital encounters in the attempt to create totally self-controlled beings, capable of spending nights and nights alone, just talking to their computers, their mind focused on nothing but the screen.
>
> (Federici, 2020/2023, p. 153)

This concerns the political erasure of the sexual. Is this where we find the lack or the excess of biopolitical management of the posthuman human? Is there, in fact, a potentially subversive sexual desire being manipulated, controlled, and separated by capital? We shall return to this topic shortly.

It is important to emphasize here the care needed to avoid completely demonizing internet hyperconnection. For Macaron, this has been and continues to be the main way of forming bonds with the Other. But at the same time, Cosenza (2022/2024) suggests that this is a threshold at which it is clinically necessary to distinguish when hyperconnection is a radical rupture with the Other. From our traditional perspective, we observe Macaron alternating between forming bonds and breaking with the Other. But here, the Other is a representative of alterity. What would be the place of alterity from a posthumanist perspective? In Lacanian theory, the Other must reveal its lack, its incompleteness, and thereby enable the emergence of the lacking and divided subject who can form bonds. In posthumanism, let us recall that the nomadic subject is relational, a branch of complexity theory that continuously emphasizes the radicality of transformation. We are in different fields, with different points of departure.

In Cosenza, there is no optimistic solution for Macaron. Hyperconnection fits into the formula of the paradigm that characterizes the pathologies of excess: *disconnection from the Other / hyperconnection to the object*, that is, a double process of

> disconnection from the symbolic Other, from the signifying operation of the laws of speech and language, from the dialectical dimension of life; and hyperconnection with the imperative of *jouissance* that invades the body of the speaking being, plunging it into an irresistible and limitless experience that repeats itself, with effects of the eclipse of the subject and devastation.
>
> (Cosenza, 2022/2024, p. 143, our translation)

The Clinical Practice

Our challenge is to consider what can be done in this scenario. We understand that there is a material world and a virtual world, and both are extremely important; both are realities. It is no longer accurate to claim there is an escape into the virtual. It is merely another way of experiencing the world; it is real. This was the turning point in our work when we sought to understand at what moment the virtual enables bonds and the formation of the bodily Self and of gender conceived from another perspective.

Working with young psychologists and psychoanalysts in training, we entered the virtual world. Our team is large, and many of these young psychologists are familiar with the games, internet language, and anime characters. We reflected on the enormous generational gap – between parents and children – regarding cultural life. Books, music, and entertainment references differ greatly and change at an incredibly fast pace. Older generations of psychoanalysts (as well as parents and grandparents) seem to have difficulty or less interest in keeping up with these changes; however, younger generations of psychologists and psychoanalysts still manage to.

The parents of these adolescents seem to have no idea what their children think, what they watch, what they know, or what they desire. In contrast, we found in manga, anime, and games bridges through which to enter the world of these young individuals, encouraging them to expand their discourse and speak about themselves. It is through these media that they construct their genders, fantasies, and desires.

What is sought in the clinic of gendered technosubjectivities? The title of Federici's work (2020/2023) suggests rethinking, redoing, and reclaiming the body under contemporary capitalism, especially in the aftermath of the COVID-19 pandemic, whose degree of impact on new subjectivities we have yet to measure. Reflecting on our patients, is there truly a stolen body? A captured sexual desire? This is undoubtedly one way to conceive of things. It is not a matter of using the body to celebrate an essentialist and biologizing discourse, which has legitimized oppression based on a supposed "human nature," but rather, in its name, to reclaim the erogenous, instinctual, and desiring aspect of the relationship with the Other.

Nearly ten years after publishing *The Posthuman*, Braidotti wrote *Posthuman Feminism* (2022), in which she locates her idea of an embodied sexuality that takes into account the materiality of bodies and their social, political, and subjective inscriptions.

Braidotti first asks whether the emphasis on technological mediation and the enhancement of the human being may have marginalized or eliminated the material bodies of human beings. Her philosophical proposal affirms that the answer is negative, even though today's bodies have been transformed into complex relational nodes. The paradigm of the nature–culture *continuum* gives way to the human–non-human bodies *continuum*, including animal life (*zoe*) in its diversity, grounded "on an endangered planet (*geo*)" and immersed in technological mediation (*techno*) (Braidotti, 2022, p. 18).

> Hence the assemblage of what I call "*zoe*/geo/technobodies." I see this approach as a critical form of de-naturalization. Bodies are neither natural nor cultural but in constant process between them, as a heterogeneous assemblage of complex relational components.
>
> (Braidotti, 2022, p. 18)

This framework allows us to look at Macaron and conceive of a body that includes the screen with all its characters, transcending the human–machine boundary, because this dichotomy has been undone. Readers should not think that the transformation we have enacted in the understanding of Macaron's body is some sort of private "intergalactic journey." We have attempted to show that Braidotti, drawing on Haraway, makes this reading possible. But perhaps it is necessary to make Braidotti's position explicit once again, and this is relatively simple. Let us take a series of questions she poses:

> What happens indeed when the traditional notion of the body as a bound and specified entity explodes into a web of human and non-human components? What happens when the skin is no longer the firm boundary of the body, but rather reveals its true nature as a porous membrane that is open onto the outside world? What if the body, in addition to perceiving, storing and retrieving flows of information and sensorial data by itself, can also be accelerated through technological enhancement?
>
> (Braidotti, 2022, p. 149)

The answers are liberating: the construction of the body, as proposed by Braidotti, collapses sexual differences and gender roles based on visually identifiable anatomical and physiological variations among sexes, races, and species. From this emerge multiple possibilities for constructing alternative bodies (Braidotti, 2022, p. 155). The binary gender system loses its meaning. The distinction between gender and body dissolves.

However, one element stands out: Braidotti emphasizes the importance of Eros – not an Eros captured and limited by sexual and gender binarism, but an Eros as an elemental force, as the centre of multiple sexed becomings. Eros, or sexuality, is the only way to understand the profound vitality and unity of living matter, approaching sexuality as both human and non-human. Sexuality, she will say, "as a trans-corporeal, enfleshed nexus, facilitates the pleasures and the dangers of the interconnections between humans and non-humans" (2022, p. 184). It is independent of reproductive politics, as Haraway had already affirmed when she stated that the cyborg was uncoupled from heterosexism and organic reproduction (Haraway, 1985/2009, p. 36).

Returning to our question: if binary gender and sexuality framed within heterosexist and reproductive norms are no longer goals to be reached in an analysis, what path should we take with Macaron? We consider as a first step the identification by us (analyst and therapeutic companion) and by Macaron that there is Eros in operation. A subversive Eros that does not meet traditional and social expectations of body and gender, but nevertheless produces bonds. Where there is desire, there is a bond. What matters is understanding that desire is situated in the Macaron *zoe/geo/technobody* and their technosubjectivity, and is addressed, at this moment, to the therapeutic companion *zoe/geo/technobody*. As Braidotti says, there is no way of knowing what posthuman desiring bodies can do.

We believe that what posthumanism allows us in this particular case of Macaron is to escape a diagnosis of pathology *avant la lettre*, while also pushing us to the limit of understanding the other as a "same." It is an exercise in radicality, in absolute alterity, perhaps even the most intimate exercise of analysis, albeit one that is no longer characterized as such in the case in question. Contrary to the famous phrase by Terence, "*Homo sum; humani nil a me alienum puto*," which translates as "I am human, and *nothing that is human is strange to me*," we could say: "I am posthuman, and everything posthuman is strange to me."

Notes

1 The critique of Jacques Lacan's notion of the symbolic as a dimension immune to social transformations was likewise undertaken by Judith Butler. For this debate, see *Psychoanalysis and Gender: Deconstructing Pathologies with Judith Butler* (Patricia Porchat, 2014, Curitiba: Editora Juruá).

2 We chose a fictitious name to protect the identity of our patient, but we believe the meaning has been preserved. The sweet can be associated with a childlike world, in which gender is less invoked than in adolescence. His parents continued using the male name assigned at birth, and he stated that he was not bothered by it. The

fact that Macaron did not wish to adopt a female name left us uncertain about how to refer to him. We have opted here for the masculine pronoun.

3 Name given to Japanese cartoons that have become increasingly popular in the Western world. We have observed that the majority of our adolescent patients watch these Japanese series quite regularly, beginning to consume them even excessively, as is the case of Macaron.

References

Ayouch, T. (2019). *Psicanálise e hibridez: Gênero, colonialidade e subjetivações*. Ed. Calligraphie.

Braidotti, R. (2013). *The posthuman*. Polity Press.

Braidotti, R. (2022). *Posthuman feminism*. Polity Press.

Cosenza, D. (2024). *Clínica do excesso: Derivas pulsionais e soluções sintomáticas na psicopatologia contemporânea*. Scriptum. (Original work published in 2022)

Deleuze, G., & Guattari, F. (1977). Anti-Oedipus. *Capitalism and Schizophrenia*. New York: Viking Press/Richard Seaver.

Espinoza, B. (2007). *Ética*. Autêntica Editora. (Original work published in 1677)

Federici, S. (2023). *Além da pele: Repensar, refazer e reivindicar o corpo no capitalismo contemporâneo* (J. P. Dias, Trans.). Elefante. (Original work published in 2020)

Ferrando, F. (2013). Posthumanism, transhumanism, antihumanism, metahumanism, and new materialisms: Differences and relations. *Existenz, 8*(2), 26–32.

Guerreiro, A. (2018). Rosi Braidotti: Para acabar de vez com as identidades. In T. Tadeu (Ed.), *Electra: Volume 3. Turismo: mobilização total*. Fundação EDP. Accessed December 14, 2024 from https://electramagazine.fundacaoedp.pt/editions/edicao-3/rosi-braidotti-para-acabar-de-vez-com-identidades

Haraway, D. (2009). Manifesto ciborgue. In T. Tadeu (Ed.), *Antropologia do ciborgue: as vertigens do pós-humano* (2nd ed.). Autêntica Editora. (Original work published in 1985)

Lacan, J. (1998). *Escritos*. Jorge Zahar.

Senso Tower. (2021). *Avakin life – Mundo virtual 3D – Overview – Google Play Store*. Accessed on December 8, 2024, from https://sensortower.com/android/br/lockwood-publishing-ltd/app/avakin-life-mundo-virtual-3d/com.lockwood-publishing.avakinlife/overview

8 The Cyborg Condition Under Realist Scrutiny

Helena Maldonado Goti

Long after Donna Haraway first published her *Manifesto for Cyborgs* in English in 1985, the statement "We are all cyborgs" still reverberates on the invisible walls of our neoliberal cybernetic society. Since then, the world has taken many turns; not all of them fortunate. Not only did we live through a pandemic that took the lives of millions of people and kept us in a lockdown for nearly two years, but also we find ourselves in the midst of an unprecedented crisis, due to climate change. In addition, the neoliberal market is increasingly voracious and unequal, the hectic race between China and the United States in terms of AI development seems unstoppable, and the number of armed conflicts so far this year 2024 is enough to depress even the most stoic. All of these elements seem to prove Nick Land's thesis that capitalism is its self-destruction.

The list could go on, but it is not my intention to foster despair; yet I will not deny the horror of living in the twilight of the modern capitalist world – quite the contrary. I intend to take a realistic position, distant from denial and despair, but deeply committed to the current situation and to the problems we face in our practice on a daily basis. In this article, I will develop the two forms of realism that I find most productive: the realism in Nick Land and in Jacques Lacan. I will explore their bases, their similarities, and their disagreements, in order to demonstrate that going back to Haraway's *Manifesto*, through the lens of the realisms of Land and Lacan, will allow us to think of a type of cyborg slightly different from Haraway's.

Psychoanalysis is a field that requires a type of labour that fluctuates at different levels. It not only requires work in intellectual terms, but fundamentally a type of labour that can only be achieved under the terms of analytic experience. And for that purpose, I find it indispensable to give an account of how the psychoanalytical experience comes to an end – not only so that it is possible to occupy the place of the analyst as a function but also as a way to fundament the purpose of the experience itself. This does not mean that experience is something that we can accumulate as if it were flying hours, although it may take many years to finish the experience.

DOI: 10.4324/9781003783862-12

Since it is so hard to determine what exactly happens within the psychoanalytical experience so that it comes to an end, the psychoanalytical field tends to be somewhat hermetic in comparison to other fields; however, in order to keep the psychoanalytical practice alive, it seems to me necessary to establish a dialogue with other fields and other paradigms. We are always at risk of losing contact with the contemporary world and succumbing to the inertia of repeating the same referents in an endogamic and self-destructive manner. Nevertheless, the history of psychoanalysis gives meaning to our practice (I am referring to the discussions that have arisen around the reading of Freud and the different currents that have derived from it), and the different authors, beginning with Freud himself, were touched by the enigmas of the practice; they dedicated their entire lives to building a solid base that would give psychoanalysis a serious status. However, it is also necessary to take into account the context of our referents, since it is always changing. That is actually the reason why the same thing that at some point constituted the very sense of our practice also arrives at a moment when it becomes an obstacle. Let us not forget that the practice of psychoanalysis in its origins made room for those things that did not make any sense – that did not fit into any knowledge.

The concept of meaning cannot only be criticized within the psychoanalytical practice; authors such as Baudrillard have pointed out that since the birth of cybernetics, our reality began to suffer from an excess of meaning.

> I call integral reality to the perpetration on the world of an unlimited operative project: that everything becomes real, that everything becomes visible and transparent, that everything is liberated, that everything is carried out and that everything has a meaning (however, what is proper to meaning is that not everything has it).
>
> (Baudrillard, 2008, p. 11)

The notion of excess is also a constant within Land's philosophy, but in terms of acceleration – that is, as a temporal structure of the accumulation of capital. In Lacan, on the other hand, we find a critique of meaning, a quest that does not accept meaning as an effect of understanding. Both authors agree that civilizations under the European capitalist model are subjected to an excess. This point is particularly explored by Land:

> Repression always fails, but nowhere is there a more variegated example of such failure than in the pretense of burying death quietly on the outskirts of the city and getting down to business. There is nothing but the historically buried layers of zero under the clay, distilling death to its ultimate liquidity, and maximizing its powers of infiltration. Marx noted this process of seepage in *Capital*, where he says: "it does not simply disappear by spilling out of the circuit of metamorphosis of a

> given commodity. Rather it constantly rushes into new places within the arena of circulation dislodged by other commodities." Dead labor is much more difficult to control than living material was; and for this reason, the Enlightenment project of burying Gothic superstition was indeed the royal road to the first truly vampiric civilization in which only death rules.
>
> (Land, 2021, p. 78)

Land's critiques provoke and revitalize contemporary philosophy and open perspectives with which to think about our practice. Lacan, on the other hand, insisted on the necessity to formalize the end of the psychanalytical experience in order to specify what kind of experience psychoanalysis is; in that sense, he also revitalized the practice by stripping it of its enlightened stability.

Regardless of all the above, Haraway's *Manifesto*, besides the fact that it remains an important reference today, it stands as a light that illuminates those parts darkened under the European civilization project. It does not deal precisely with the consequences of the development of technology, but it shows that through its development emerges the hybridity of our condition. At the same time, it opens a way to destabilize identities and question the concept of "humanity." This concept, in fact, had already been the object of fierce criticism before Haraway, since structuralism found a way to think in terms of relationships and not so much in terms of elements within a totality, or even in terms of identities. But it is with Haraway that social identities definitely lose meaning.

> Identities seem contradictory, partial and strategic, gender, race and class, with the recognition of their historical and social constitutions won after long struggles is not enough to provide the "essential" basis of belief. There is nothing in the fact of "being a woman" that naturally unites women. There is not even the state of "being" a woman.
>
> (Haraway, 1995, p. 264)

In psychoanalysis, structuralism also made itself present thanks to Jacques Lacan, who took the liberty of reading Sigmund Freud through several other authors who were outside the field of psychoanalysis, one of them being Claude Lévi-Strauss. But even before being so strongly influenced by structuralism and linguistics, Lacan had already pointed out in 1936 something similar to what Haraway raised in her *Manifesto*, but in the context of the question of the configuration of subjectivity. The central idea of Lacan's paper, which was later published as a text (Lacan, 2006), is that the ego (*je*) is constructed from the outside and so its nature is orthopaedic. The totality of the form found in the notion of the ego (*je*) is sustained in the perception of the image that is first presented to the infant in the mirror, and which functions as an alienating armature that marks its rigid structure in the mental development.

Unlike Freud, who preserves in his way of approaching the psychic apparatus the idea of the proto-ego, subjectivity from the Lacanian point of view – because it is orthopaedic – is in a way, since the beginning of its very own foundations, cyborg. Not in the sense of a coupling between machines and organisms, but in the sense that it configurates itself from an exteriority mediated by a very precarious type of technology, if you will, but technology at the end of the day. The point being, the importance of technology in our time, particularly with the emergence of smart devices. Such technology introduced a different kind of orthopaedics, mounted on a subjectivity that, according to Lacan, is already in itself torn due to its external configuration. Like Haraway, Lacan would argue that it is precisely through technology that the hybrid condition of subjectivity unfolds.

Moreover, we could consider following Land – who, inspired by authors such as Baudrillard (2005) and his idea of integral reality and by Deleuze and Guattari (2000) and their notion of deterritorialization – affirms that we are actually exposed to it on a daily basis. The constant flow of information, which in turn produces subjects, shows in a forceful but also problematic way the orthopaedic nature of subjectivity to which we referred earlier with Lacan. The effects of the use of social networks, insofar as they are designed to create a "fictitious" identity that generates addiction among users (Seymour, 2019) and strengthens the fiction of the ego, also dissolve or destabilize the boundaries established by the enlightenment paradigm between fiction and reality. Land, for example wrote: "under teleopoetic direction, ontological dualism is dissociated from the present, rendering increasingly obsolete the question of what is real" (Land, 2021). As a matter of fact, the development of technology in the field of cybernetics and the internet inaugurated a very specific kind of hyperreality. Its systematic use fosters a very peculiar kind of hyperrealism.

In the face of this hyperreal condition, Lacan's and Land's realisms operate as tools of resistance because, even though they agree in granting a place of truth to fiction, they also generate a critique of humanism and anthropocentrism which is inherent to the project of Enlightenment. Something that we do not find in the transhumanist proposals, which are unable to go beyond such a paradigm; they actually perpetuate it (Ferrando, 2019). But let us slow down a bit, because even though Nick Land is a well-known philosopher within certain fields, within the field of psychoanalysis, very few people know who he is.

Nick Land and Speculative Realism

Speculative realism is a contemporary philosophical current whose origins can be traced to a conference held in the UK in 2007, attended by Quentin

Meillassoux, Iain Hamilton Grant, Graham Harman, and Ray Brassier. Since then, each of these authors has developed various forms of realism. However, they are united by the critique of Kantian idealism in terms of the consequences that remain at the epistemological level regarding access to reality or access to the real. Let us remember that from the Kantian epistemology, the thing-in-itself is strictly inaccessible. We only have access to what the conditions of possibility of reason allow us to access. That is to say, knowledge is always a kind of network constructed from the conditions of possibility of reason; speculative realism seeks alternatives to overcome the correlation between thought and being, between subject and object, which derive from this idealism. Thus, they consider that the real exists as such, independently of the existence of human reason; some of them, like Meillassoux, argue that speculation is the form of access to this absolute real. This means that they do not always agree on the nature of the real, as well as its access.

Within speculative realism, we find different currents associated with certain authors. For example, object-oriented ontology is associated with Graham Harman and accelerationism with Nick Land. This latter one characterizes, according to our author, acceleration:

> As a historical phenomenon tied to capitalism, but also as a concomitant and creative process linked to the regeneration of culture, cybernetics and the philosophy of technology, and ultimately linked to the inertia of a cosmic process that tends irrevocably towards its acceleration and disintegration.
>
> (Land, 2021, p. 10)

According to Land's book Teleoplexy (2023), Land is a philosopher who was deeply influenced by the developments of cybernetics, particularly the approaches of Norbert Wiener, but also by Gilles Deleuze, Félix Guattari, George Bataille, and Jean-François Lyotard and, last but not least, by science fiction and horror.

Land's approaches are of such a radical nature that they necessarily lead to an anti-humanism which dismisses any political and philosophical project that attempts to vindicate the concept of humanity. This is similar to the way in which Lacan distanced himself from humanism when, in *Science and Truth,* he wrote: "It is well known that I have always been repugnant to the appellation of human sciences, which seems to me to be the very call of servitude" (Lacan, 1975, p. 838).

For Land, there is no possibility for progress; as a matter of fact, it never existed, just as in Lacan's criticism of historicism in psychoanalysis:

> It is to state sufficiently, in passing, that in psychoanalysis history is a dimension distinct from that of development, and that this aberration attempts to reduce it to that dimension. History does not proceed

> except against the backdrop of development. A point from which history as a science can perhaps take advantage, if it wants to escape the ever-present threat of a providential conception of its course.
>
> (Lacan, 1975, p. 846)

But the most interesting thing about Land, from my point of view, is that he considers horror as the only true end of philosophy. Land finds affinity in the literature of H.P. Lovecraft and Edgar Allan Poe, which dives into a different kind of horror, radically different from fear or terror. It is the horror of the unknown:

> Horror is inseparable from a specific task: to create an object of the unknown, as unknown. Only in these terms can its essential achievements be assessed.
>
> Isolating the abstract purpose of horror, therefore, does not require a supplementary philosophical operation. Horror defines itself through a pact with abstraction, a compulsion so primordial that disciplined metaphysics can barely, and always belatedly, strive to recapture it . . . Horror is the first to find "that" which philosophy ultimately craves to know.
>
> (Land, 2012, p. 44)

It is inevitable, for those of us dedicated to psychoanalysis, not to find in this paragraph a clear resonance with the notion of the *unheimlich* – a term that was translated into Spanish by Etcheverry as the ominous, as Freud worked it in his 1919 text – and here is where some potentially productive ties between Land's accelerationism and psychoanalysis can be explored.

While Freud's proposal is to make room for the repressed unconscious that returns from the outside and appears as alien, but familiarly foreign or strange, authors such as Mark Fisher, a disciple of Land, rather emphasize the power of the slippage of the *unheimlich* (which preserves a link with the familiar) towards the eerie, which is detached from any relationship with the known.

> The eerie has to do with the most fundamental metaphysical questions that can be asked; questions related to existence and non-existence, why is there something when there shouldn't be anything, why is there nothing when there should be something?
>
> (Fisher, 2016, p. 15)

For Fisher, the eerie is in consonance with Lacan's *jouissance*, precisely because *jouissance* is the terrain of the unknowable. Nevertheless, the question is complex. On the one hand, the repressed unconscious, strictly speaking, according to Freud, is unknowable. On the other hand, Freud ends up resorting, as Fisher says, to the concept of castration to explain the *unheimlich* – something that Fisher bitterly reproaches him for. As always, Freud, while opening an unprecedented breach, on the other hand returns to the terrain of that which is knowable.

With Lacan, the question becomes a little more akin to the interests of Land and the CCRU group, because structuralism and linguistics allow him to approach Descartes very differently; thus, he was able to forge his peculiar subject. This is a subject in opposition to the ego, which can be detached from the Cartesian *cogito*, since the "I think" is divided into a subject of the enunciation and a subject of the statement. That is to say, the one who reads the sentence versus the one who is grammatically included in the sentence. This leads us to the fact that there is no subject beforehand; there is no thinking subject who can guarantee existence. When the phrase "I think" is said, not only is it possible to state that the subject is the effect of thought and not the other way around – with which Descartes would not disagree so much – but it is also plausible to raise the question of who exactly is this ego that thinks? Finally, it also brings the possibility to highlight the distance from existence. Hence, Lacan reads Descartes' phrase changing the comma, and in doing so, he prioritizes existence over thought: *I think therefore, I am.*

The approach is akin to Land because speculative realisms also seek a subjectivity without an individual who thinks. The fact that the subject is the effect of the unconscious – and not the other way around – makes the egotistic decentring become a common ground.

> In a word, we will find here again the subject of the signifier as we articulated it last year. Transported by the signifier in his relation to the signifier-other, he must be severely distinguished both from the biological individual and from any psychological evolution subsumable as a subject of the understanding.
>
> (Lacan, 1975, p. 854)

Lacan carefully reforms and proposes a different way to practise psychoanalysis; it diminishes the role of interpretation. His proposal departs from his three registers (Imaginary, Symbolic, and Real) as a starting point. His teaching is not homogeneous, and there are moments where he is more inclined towards one register or the other. In first instance – and only in retrospect – we could say that he begins by exploring the register of the imaginary with the mirror stage and paranoid psychosis (Aimée's thesis), but very soon the emphasis turns towards the function of speech and language in the analytic experience; this is the Lacan that most people know, at least in Latin America. However, his journey does not stop there, and in his last seminars he leans towards the register of the real. In doing so, the affinities with speculative realism become more evident. In the case of Lacan's reading of the role of castration, for example, it is not a matter of conceiving it as a return to that which is knowable, as Fisher's critique of Freud points out, but it can be conceived as the limit of the phallic logic, which is in the place of the Other. That is to say, each sex (male or female exclusively – here is the binarism in Lacan) is played out in relation to the other sex, which at this moment (the seminar *Of a discourse other than that of the semblant*) is the Other. And there is something of the real, of the real of sexual *jouissance* in the phallus. Lacan says:

> We must say it, all that was enunciated to us as the spring of the unconscious represents nothing more than the horror of that truth . . . It is not something particularly pleasant to hear, it is what is usually packaged under the rubric of the castration complex.
>
> (Lacan, 2006)

But let us explore some other affinities and problematics between Land's and Lacan's realism.

Truth and Fiction

The way in which Lacan goes about configuring his subject, beginning with the Freudian formations of the unconscious and Descartes' *Metaphysical Meditations*, allows him later to draw a division between knowledge and truth.

In the text *The Science and the Truth* (1966), Lacan maintains a tension between science and psychoanalysis based on subject and truth. Paradoxically, the subject on which psychoanalysis operates is the subject of science (Lacan, 2006). As we said, this way of approaching the subject is only possible because of the singular reading he maintains of Descartes's subject; however, as far as truth is concerned, it does mark an important difference: while in science it is taken as a cause in its formal aspect, in psychoanalysis it is a cause in its material aspect. Lacanian materialism is a materialism of the signifier. We could say that it is a realism articulated from the signifier which stretches on to the real. The text starts from the canonical idea that the unconscious is language, although language is not reduced to words, but it maintains a close relationship with it. Instead of thinking of truth as something that is found at the end of the road – that is, as a consequence of speaking – it is a matter of how truth is founded on the basis of speaking. That is why Lacan insists on saying "I, the truth, speak . . . ." It is truth that speaks in itself without ever landing in a firm and well-defined territory, because the only thing that can be said of truth is that there is no Other of the Other.

> It means, beyond the allegory that all that is to be said of truth, of the only one, namely that there is no metalanguage, that no language could say the truth of the true, since truth is founded by the fact that it speaks, and since it has no other means to do so.
>
> (Lacan, 1966, p. 846)

And yet, truth is related to the unnameable and, at the same time, it has little in common with the Kantian noumenon. In any case, as he well said in the session of February 17, 1971: "Everything that depends on the effect of language, everything that establishes the *demansion* of truth, is posited on the basis of a fictional structure" (Lacan, 2025). So truth is not unknowable, and it maintains a relationship with the subject.

Demansion is a neologism created by Lacan to designate the place of the Other of truth; it contains the word *mansion*, which in French means "house." In this seminar – dedicated to the nature of the discourse of the analyst, which is a discourse that is not of the semblant – he devotes himself to treating the difference between writing and language. The nature of the mansion (the house) of language can only be questioned by the written – that is, by logical writing – but the written is only constituted by its reference to language.

The Non-Sexual Relation

The difference between writing and language leads to the approach of the non-sexual relation, which is the turning point where knowledge and truth meet. Perhaps, in order to discuss this idea, it is necessary to point out a nuance that consists in the fact that, in French, there are two words for relation. The first one, relation, has the same meaning as in English, but the second one, rapport, has a mathematical meaning. Lacan uses the word *rapport*. So, the problem of the non-relation is, in principle, a mathematical problem that designates the impossibility of a mathematically relationship between two different elements – a and b, for example. In such a way, man and woman in the formulas of sexuation fulfil in Lacan, first, a mathematical function, and only later a function of alterity. It is about the Other as the other sex.

> Sexual identification does not consist in believing oneself to be a man or a woman, but in taking into account that there are women, for the boy, that there are men, for the girl. And what matters is not even so much what they experience, it is a real situation, allow me. For men, the girl is the phallus, and it is what emasculates them. For women, the boy is the same thing, the phallus, and this is what emasculates them too because they only get one penis, and that is failed. Neither the boy nor the girl is at risk in the first place except for the dramas they unleash, they are the phallus for a moment.
>
> (Lacan, 1971, p. 33)

The question then is that man and/or woman are positions to be taken towards the Other – that is, signifiers. However, these signifiers are loaded with cultural constructs from where they were actually gestated in the first place. This generates a great confusion because then, what are we talking about? Strictly speaking, at this point in Lacan's teaching, the Other – as another sex – harbours something of the impossibility of sex. As Lina Rovira says in her text on the formulas of sexuation (2018):

> The subject, withdrawn in the only certainties of his phantasm, would say that he is on the defensive of confronting the limits of the signifier, in terms of the real of sex. And sex, as the place in which is situated this truth impossible to know and of which, moreover, nothing is wanted to know.
>
> (Rovira, 2018, p. 52)

The topic is extensive and requires further elaboration, but since our interest in this article is only to locate the type of realism in Lacan and Land and its consequences in terms of what Haraway has made us think, I only want to point out the real aspect of sex and the non-sexual relation. This serves to show that Lacan's realism is a realism that harbours within it that which is disturbing: the *eerie*, I would say. Thus, we can actually find a response to Fisher's critique of Freud, but one which is very far away from any of the concerns that have unfolded within gender theory, feminisms, and queer theory.

Xenofeminism, Cyberfeminism, and Queer Theory

The collective Laboria Cuboniks (2018), which has been very close to the CCRU, has proposed a feminism called Xenofeminism. Such a proposal is based on the idea of the *xeno* – that is, the foreign, the alien, the strange, but especially, the hospitable. Formed by scientists and artists who, aware of the heteronormative and patriarchal side of scientific discourse, wrote the *Xenofeminist Manifesto.*

The proposals of this collective are similar to the realisms we have been dealing with and are immersed in the difference between the realism of Land and Lacan that we just pointed out. Such a difference concerns the real of sex, the non-relation, the subject, and *jouissance*. Meanwhile, Land only refers to the absolutely unknowable, but real. As Lina Rovira says in relation to sexual difference, quoting Santiago Peidro – who studies the meeting points between psychoanalysis and queer theory:

> Queer does it (address sexual difference) from a political and sociocultural dimension and psychoanalysis from the fixations of *jouissance*, the reality of the unconscious and the structural mismatch of the sexes.
>
> (Rovira, 2018, p. 121)

On the other hand, if we go back to Haraway, we find in her *Manifesto* a mention of cyborg sex:

> It (cyborg sex) restores some of the reproductive baroque of ferns and invertebrates (magnificent organic prophylactics against heterosexuality) because their reproduction does not require coupling.
>
> (Haraway, 1995, p. 254)

Without denying the real of sex, Haraway strips it of its binarism. I wonder what Lacan would have thought of this? In fact, the *Manifesto*'s challenge is precisely a future without gender – akin to what some contemporary feminisms, such as Xenofeminism itself, defend – and a bet on an incorporation of the machinic. In that sense, also, it is a bet on a form of prosthesis that we could locate as real in the Lacanian sense of the term.

This is also the case with the cyberfeminism of Sadie Plant (2004), who centred her text "The Future looms: Weaving Women and cybernetics" on the idea of tying together the destiny of machines and women, insofar as they rebel against heteropatriarchal control. The text is interesting because it brings closer the feminist struggles and the emergence of artificial intelligences. These, as disruptive technologies, were sexed as feminine. Technologies, like women, have lived as a function of men, but Plant hopes for the development of technology – which, in her point of view, will be increasingly independent of humans – as well as the feminization of work via these new technologies. In the same way that Haraway and Lacan used technological development to show our hybrid condition, Plant considers that cyberspace confronts us with the truth of the illusory constructs of body and gender.

Now we can go weaving our way towards some type of conclusion. The realisms we have addressed inherit a series of problems that we will not be able to solve in this article. On the one hand, we have Lacan's real, which is very much present in our clinic, given that the unconscious, since its Freudian origins, has a strong foundation in the unknowable. This is the gap that Lacan opens when, in constructing his subject and his object, he tries to overcome Kantian idealism by not considering that we are dealing with the noumenon in his absolute impossibility. He put up his stakes on mathematics and topology in order to be able to scrape the real, in both its imaginary and symbolic intersections. In my point of view, this is an immense contribution, which shifts further the analytical practice towards a territory not illuminated by the paradigms of Cartesian modernity – a practice that grants a fundamental place to the real of the body, as well as to the access of the object (*petit a*). However, as we have already pointed out, the problem seems to remain on the distance that we find, for example, in the elaboration of the formulas of sexuation and the political and social aspect of the signifiers man/woman. This remains a perspective impossible to avoid, given that we live within society and gender constructs which are an intrinsic part of both our social and subjective lives, regardless of whether we distance ourselves from them or not. Yet, we cannot deny their realness. This is a problem commonly encountered among Lacanian analysts who literarily follow Lacan with a lack of critique. Some of them even consider psychoanalysis to be beyond any social context.

As for Land's realism, we can say that its power lies not only in the forcefulness of the criticisms of neoliberalism and the self-destructive aspect of capitalism but also in the fact that he commits to harbouring – in the midst of the catastrophe in which we find ourselves – horror as an unprecedented and necessary form of knowledge. There, he encounters Lacan's own reading of castration. Moreover, the accelerationism he posits is, above all, a form of time proper to capital. Yet, the fact that the form of time of capital is acceleration does not mean that it remains the only form of time. So, Land's developments are always on the horizon of quantum physics, which proposes a different time or even the non-existence of time as we conceive it. Land's realism is a realism that gives place to the future as a form of the past and to the past as a form of the future; however, when it comes to the difference of the sexes, he has little to say.

Last but not least, Haraway's cyborg – through the lens of these realisms – can now also consider this dimension of the real in both senses (Lacan's and Land's). This opens a way to show the illusory and the limitedness of our "human" condition, as well as the potency of horror as a form of knowledge.

The nature of the cyborg can now be expanded because it not only harbours the unknown as unknown, in Land's way but also the real dimension of the signifier, of sex, and of the non-relation to which Lacan appeals.

Bibliography

Baudrillard, J. (2005). *The intelligence of evil or the lucidity pact*. Bloomsbury.

Cuboniks, L. (2018). *The Xenofemenist manifesto: A politics for alienation*. Verso Books.

Deleuze, G. & Guattar, F. (2000). *A thousand plateaus: Capitalism and schizophrenia*. Bloomsbury Publishing.

Ferrando, F. (2019). *Philosophical posthumanism*. Bloomsbury.

Fisher, M. (2016). *The weird and eerie (beyond the unheimlich)*. Repeater.

Haraway, D. (2016). *Cyborg manifesto: Science, technology and socialist feminism in the late twentieth century*. University of Minnesota Press.

Lacan, J. (2006). *Écrits: The first complete edition In English*. Norton & Co.

Lacan, J. (2025). *The seminar. Book XVIII: On a discourse that might not be a semblance*. Polity Press.

Land, N. (2012). *The dark enlightenment*. Imperium Press.

Land, N. (2023, August 4). Teleoplexy. Notes on acceleration. https://www.researchgate.net/publication/32569925_Teleoplexy_Notes_on_Acceleration

Plant, S. (2004). *The future looms*. Routledge.

Rovira, L. (2018). *Sexuación y formalización. Diversas lecturas de las fórmulas de la sexuación lacanianas*. Brueghel.

Seymour, R. (2019). *The twittering machine*. The Indigo Press.

Part 4

Multiverse

The Diverse, the Multiple, the Nomadic

9 From "Who" to "What" in the Posthuman Turn

Mónica B. Cragnolini

Humanities have long been haunted by two ghosts that besiege them: the animal and the machinic (Cragnolini, 2017). The question of the posthuman – which can be traced back to the thought of Nietzsche, with his idea of the *Übermensch* (ultrahuman) as "another mode of being" (Cragnolini, 2014) as opposed to any notion of the human (and not, as has been interpreted, as a "superhuman") – points to a crisis in the idea of subjectivity that, in the 19th and early 20th centuries, has its referents in Nietzsche, Marx, and Freud. What these three "masters of suspicion" have in common, as Ricoeur has called them, is that by putting subjectivity in crisis from different perspectives, they show that "what is proper" to the human is in crisis.

The animal and the machinic haunt these pretended "own": both destabilize the baton of subjectivity, reason, and the possibility of agency. If the subject has self-positioned itself from a pretended agency, the animal (in itself and in others) makes patent that which is indomitable by such reason, as well as non-agency (for, as Nietzsche will say, "*Es denkt*", "it thinks") (Nietzsche, 1980, *KSA 5, JGB* §17, p. 31). And the machinic disturbs its supposed property of freedom (of choice, of action, of decision). Both phantoms (animal and machine) put consciousness – one of the places of settlement for "humanity" – in crisis. Animals and machines prowl that walled place of consciousness, that "little chamber", as Nietzsche (1980, *KSA* 5, *GM* III, §18, p. 383) would say and destabilize it, whether through ethological studies or the advances of artificial intelligence.

I will refer, from this interpretative context, to "another way of being" of the so-called "human" in posthumanities (i.e., our disciplines "solicited" and haunted by the ghosts indicated). The Derridean syntagm of the "transition from the *who* to the *what*" will allow me to point out the characteristics of this "other way of being".

The Transition From Who to What

Derrida (2003, pp. 257–258) has indicated that his last works can be read in the direction of the "transit from the who to the what" (and he clarifies that

DOI: 10.4324/9781003783862-14

themes such as hospitality, gift, and forgiveness are understandable in the context of such a syntagm).

Already in a volume of *Cahiers Confrontation* dedicated to the question of "who comes after the subject?", Blanchot (1989, p. 49) had questioned the question itself: why "who" comes? Why not "what is it that" comes? In this place of the what, the ghosts of the animal and the machine become visible – entities which have always been thought of as what, as *res*, as thing, as opposed to the sovereign who, producer and agent. Being considered as "what" places them at the disposal of the "who", and an authoritarian and sacrificial bond is somehow naturalized with all that is posited as "what".

But the "who" of the human and of the subject have been in crisis for a long time: what is questioned is the subject of the metaphysics of subjectivity – that which is self-positioned in the place of the self. To be "I" is to occupy a place; in this sense, the subject is an assumption of location and hierarchy, and in that positioning, it is constructed as conscious and self-conscious.

It is in these aspects of subjectivity and the human that the animal and the machinic have an impact. The machine has been haunting since the industrial revolution, but in the present age, the expansion of teletechnologies makes that autotelic, self-positioned subject only a tiny point in a network of decisions in which algorithms and commercial interests take precedence, under the simulacrum of the free decision of tastes in a multiplicity of choices. On the other hand, this mode of the human in the function of "subject" preserves the illusion of egoic self-positioning in the constant repetition of images of oneself in social networks: iterated, it pretends to be assured, recognized, and hierarchized.

As for the ghost of the animal, the critical studies of animality of the last two decades and ethology since the beginning of the 20th century put the "properly human" characteristics in crisis. When, in the 14th century, Coluccio Salutati defines the *studia humanitatis*, he indicates five disciplines as parts of it: grammar, rhetoric, poetics, history, and moral philosophy. These disciplines give an account of the property of the human – of those characteristics that could erect an exclusive "proper" of man in the face of theological studies, which subordinated everything human to a higher authority and to a limited knowledge obscured by dogmas, mysteries, and faith. It is in this confrontation of the humanities and humanism with theological studies that it is necessary to understand the place of the hierarchical self-positioning of the self, which comes to replace God as the centre of the real and to take his place. This "proper" of the human implied that everything that was not "properly" human was part of that world that could be appropriated by man: "things" over which he could exercise his dominion. The "who" can thus be erected, in an appropriating manner, over all "what": humans not considered "who" (those deprived of rights: migrants, trafficked persons) and non-humans: animals and the whole earth, thought of as a resource at the service of the existing human. When everything is at man's disposal, the relationship between property on an ontological level (as an attribute of the human existent) and property in a material and concrete sense becomes evident: it is possible to be the owner of everything real to the extent that one is a subject – that is, an entity autotelically erected as the purpose of everything that exists. This self-erection founds a structural violence with respect to everything living – a violence that is often not perceived as such because it is naturalized that the place of the human is found in this centrality and possibility of dominion over everything that *is*. This naturalization makes an alliance with the moral question, insofar as it is considered that "human dignity" is what allows differentiating the "person" (the juridical way of understanding the subject) from the thing, including the animal in that category.

But neither language, nor the memory present in history, nor the creation of poetics, nor morality, are today considered exclusively human attributes. Therefore, rather than humanities, we should speak of posthumanities, haunted by the animal and the machinic.

The double phantasm of the animal and the machinic found its perfect form of conjuration in the idea of the *bête-machine*, which is constituted in the 16th century from the work of Pereira (2000)[1] and which would later be taken up again by the followers of Descartes. The figure of the animal–machine is very suggestive, since it locates in a single entity the two fears of siege of the human itself that we are analysing: the fear of the machine – more efficient, faster, and with more power, speed, constancy, and operative capacity than the human existent – and the fear of the animal, the haunting limit of the cultural. The derivations of the animal–machine theory allow us to understand many political and social issues that were at stake at a time when the advance of colonialism required philosophical (and theological) arguments to justify the extermination of native peoples and the slave trade.

How can the fear of the machinic and the animal be conjured up today? The model of the *bête machine* is still present, despite all the ethological studies that have shown that suffering, language, creation, the formation of techniques, and so many characteristics that were considered to be exclusive to humans are also characteristics of non-human animals. The idea that the living animal is a reaction machine is naturalized: this gives an alibi, even to the right-thinking, for the massive and industrial use of animals that are produced (made to be born) only to die – that is, animals whose reason for coming to life is to die to satisfy the needs of the human animal, with which they are already always dead. Animals would not be slaughtered if it were admitted that they are alive, feel, and have language – even though it is known. Animals would not be used in scientific experimentation if it were admitted that they suffer and that they have interests – in spite of the fact that it is known.

In other words, the animal is transformed into a machine to prevent the ghost of its suffering image: most carnivores cover their ears when they hear about the suffering of the animal – now a corpse on their plate – ready to be consumed.

The other ghost – that of the machine – how can it be conjured up? In Alan Turing's test, the machine had to convince the human; today, humans must convince machines that we are indeed human. We must "prove" to machines that we are not machines (that is the function of *captcha – Completely Automated Public to tell Computers and Humans Apart*). On the other hand, artificial intelligence manages to perform activities that were always considered "properly human", such as, for example, creativity in play, eroding those "proper" human cognitive capacities: the possibility of representation, consciousness, autonomy, and the possibility of choice.

These two haunters – animal and machine – cannot be confronted in the fields of humanities from the conjuration and negation (propitiating, e.g., returns to humanisms), but from the possibility of thinking politics of hospitality with the ghosts that haunt the notion of subject. The notion of subjectivity harbours the remnants of the uncontamination implied by the idea of the sovereign subject, which is why it is necessary to rethink this notion from contemporary issues, such as the ideas of otherness and community.

How can we be hospitable to these ghosts? In the first place, it is no longer possible to continue naturalizing the idea that to be a subject is to be sacrificial – that is to say, devouring, phagocytizing, and introjecting otherness. For this, we must recognize that the sacrificed bodies of animals in the productive chain are also the sacrificed bodies of humans considered "animals" in the nature–culture distinction – a distinction that is maintained to the extent that culture continues to be thought of as the possibility of "making human" all that is natural, as available for that "humanity" that is forged, then, from the sacrifice of the vital. Along with animals, the bodies most available for sacrifice are those of women and children, subjected to trafficking and abuse in an almost "naturalised" way.

Secondly, we should no longer propose a dignity of the human from that self-erected place of the subject: to be hospitable to the stranger implies not only accepting the contamination of the different (animals, machines) but also assuming the responsibility and (if you will allow me the much-detested term, "guilt") of the sacrifice of the living. The mode of being of the posthuman (that which is traversed by the machinic, but also by the living assumed as such) is not the aseptic and sovereign subject, but a depowered, vulnerable mode that assumes the fragility of all that is living and, with it, the care it deserves.

Thus, I point out again, it is necessary to be hospitable to these two phantoms, instead of conjuring them up and denying them as dangers to our pretended self-conscious subjectivity. In the issue of *Cahiers Confrontation* which I mentioned earlier, Blanchot – faced with the question of what comes after the subject – mentions modes such as the Nietzschean ultrahuman, the Heideggerian *Ereignis*, Nancy's demand for the inoperative community, or the strangeness of Lévinas's absolute Other: all four modes of a detachment of subjectivity with respect to its attributes (those attributes that transform it into dignity and sovereignty).

The Nietzschean ultrahuman was Nietzsche's posthuman proposal, jaded and disgusted by the "human, all too human". The current pandemic has made it clear how miserable the human way of being is in its subjugation of the planet and other forms of life: we are about to forget what we questioned last year, when we warned about the problem of zoonotic diseases and all that they implied as a consequence of the intensive animal production chain – at the level of soil erosion, climate change, deforestation, and so forth (Cragnolini, 2020). We are about to consider that we have defeated something through immunization and vaccines; we are about to resume our usual arrogance of thinking that we can destroy everything and that later science – which helped us to destroy – will help us (now, with vaccines) to continue doing what we used to do.

Thinking our posthumanity in the pandemic implies recognizing that defenestration of the "who" does not attempt against any dignity of the human, and it does attempt against the dignity of other forms of life to continue in that subjugating self-positioning of otherness that is the subject. Man, as Nietzsche thought, can no longer be preserved (this is the position of humanism) or improved (the thesis of transhumanism). The pandemic has shown us that we can no longer "live from" or "live against": it is time to understand how to "live with".

Note

1 Gómez Pereira (2000) stated in 1554 that animals lack sentience. If animals felt, then humans who use them for work, expose them to danger, and force them to carry heavy loads would not be "good." In this regard, see Cragnolini (2015).

References

Blanchot, M. (1989). Qui. *Cahiers Confrontation*, *20*(1989), 49–51.

Cragnolini, M. B. (2014). An 'other way of being'. The Nietzschean animal: Contributions to the question of biopolitic. In V. Lemm (Ed.), *Nietzsche and the becoming of life* (pp. 214–230). Fordham University Press.

Cragnolini, M. B. (2015). Animula, vagula, blandula, o sobre el alma perdida de los animales. *Lo Sguardo*, *18*(2015_II), 317–329.

Cragnolini, M. B. (2017). Animales y máquinas entre el quién y el qué. In M. B. Cragnolini (Ed.), *"Quién" o "qué". Los tránsitos del pensar actual hacia la comunidad de los vivientes* (pp. 7–14). La Cebra.

Cragnolini, M. B. (2020). Ontología de guerra frente a las zoonosis. In *AA.VV., La fiebre* (pp. 39–48). ASPO.

Derrida, J. (2003). As if it were possible. Within such limits. In *Papel máquina*. Trotta.

Gómez Pereira, A. (2000). *Antoniana margarita*. Facsimile reproduction of the edition of 1749, preliminary study and Spanish version of J. L. Barreiro Barreiro. Compostela-Oviedo.

Nietzsche, F. (1980). *Sämtliche Werke. Kritische Studienausgabe in 15 Bänden*. Walter de Gruyter/Deutsche Taschenbuch Verlag (Cited as *KSA*, previously indicating the work according to the acronym proposed by the edition, then the volume of the *KSA*, then the corresponding paragraph or part, and finally the page).

10 The Polyphonic Subjectivities of Posthumanism

María Luisa Silva Checa

First Chords

My engagement with posthumanist theories evokes in me a mix of excitement and unease. Curiously, these are the same emotions mentioned by Rosi Braidotti – one of the leading voices in the field – in *The Posthuman Knowledge* (2019). I feel excited because these theories offer an opportunity to expand our horizon of understanding regarding what we are living through today or, at the very least, to encourage us to "think about thinking," as the philosopher François Jullien (2013, p. 11) suggests. The unease, on the other hand, stems from the realization that what these theories announce is far from a dystopian futurology: it reflects the very way we currently live.

The critical posthumanist approach advocated by Braidotti (2006, 2013) calls for a profound revision of humanism in order to face the challenges posed by advanced industrial capitalism and its culture of communications, biotechnologies, cybercultures, and the new subjectivities emerging from these transformations – including new forms of gender and eroticism. This directly challenges psychoanalysts: it demands that we rethink our theories and explore how these posthuman complexities traverse the processes of subjectivation. Only in doing so will we be able to refine our clinical instruments and listen, with greater precision, to the musicality of contemporary clinical work. In this way, we take part in a broader challenge that demands a transdisciplinary polyphony.

This chapter offers a few reflections on the contributions of posthumanist thought – focusing primarily on the work of Rosi Braidotti – and explores its resonances with certain philosophical and psychoanalytic developments. Accompanying this reflection are notes drawn from the field of musical perception as a way of expanding our sensitivity to subjective processes in times of mutation.

In music, the opening chords establish an atmosphere, a kind of promise of what the melody will later develop. Analogously, I suggest that we approach contemporary phenomena as one might listen to the first

DOI: 10.4324/9781003783862-15

measures of an unfamiliar piece: with a radically open attitude, akin to analytic listening.

From my experience, approaching posthumanist theories involves a kind of recursive movement. It requires a disposition towards the unheard-of – a sensibility that allows us to apprehend what these theories seek to convey. In turn, these theories are precisely what lead us to new horizons of thought. This is perhaps the same attitude demanded by the "availability to thought" Jullien (2013) speaks of, or the capacity for wonder needed to embark on a psychoanalytic journey, as proposed by Leopoldo Nosek (2017).

Particularly inspiring to me is Janine Puget's (2020) proposal in *Vivir en desequilibrio permanente* (*Living in Permanent Imbalance*), where she posits that both analytical listening and life itself demand an open mind and a willingness to be "perforated" by the unfamiliar. This openness is essential for grasping phenomena that are already occurring but, as she warns, do not yet have names or histories.

Who are we? Where are we? Where are we going? These traditionally philosophical questions now resonate powerfully across various domains of thought. They are no longer the exclusive province of metaphysics but have become urgent tools for those seeking to understand the transformations of the world we inhabit and the subjectivities that emerge within it.

As psychoanalysts, we might begin by questioning our own stance in the face of these issues. What accounts for our apprehension towards novel thought? Why do we resist engaging with emerging ideas? Embracing this task is not a luxury, but an ethical responsibility – an imperative, especially for those of us who work with human suffering. After all, this very openness is what we encourage in our patients. We should, therefore, embody it in our own praxis.

Rigid, fixed positions do not honour the subversive and revealing impulse that once animated psychoanalysis when it sought resonances at the margins of the analytic field to better grasp psychic reality. Today, more than ever, we need a plural psychoanalysis – one that can expand towards a theory and praxis developing at the borders and interfaces: at the edges of the body, in the relation to objects and to otherness, in the dynamics of social life, and the thickness of historical context. To uphold this legacy and move in openness means resisting the pull of a narrow focus that deceptively invites us to mistake the part for the whole. When we fixate on a fragment of the picture, we forget our drive to dismantle opaque phenomena; in doing so, we operate on poorly understood syntheses, neglecting the vastness of what we do not yet know.

While psychoanalysis, like any science, requires methodological abstraction to delimit its object of study, we must not forget that such framing is a tool of the researcher – not a faithful reflection of the psychic phenomenon's complexity. A focus may help reveal detail, but it does not mean that the surrounding context is irrelevant. On the contrary, the context is a porous border in constant interdependence with other contours, operating across distinct temporalities and visibilities.

As Edgar Morin (1990/2011) proposed through his notion of complex thought, it is increasingly difficult – within the contemporary landscape of knowledge – to do without a perspective open to such complexity. Yet resistance to these changes persists, visible in the tendency to minimize or pathologize transformations that challenge established norms. Such reactions reveal a conflict between subjectivities rooted in fixed categories and the emerging forms driven by posthumanist thinking.

Sounds from Posthumanism

Opening a space to listen to the reverberations of posthumanism is no simple task. There are many possible entry points; for that reason, I will limit myself to sketching just a few.

The first point I want to emphasize in Braidotti's critical posthumanism (2019/2020, 2013/2015, 2006/2009) is her understanding of life as a continuous process of self-creation, transformation, and relationality that runs through all entities on the planet. Influences such as the Spinozist notion of a generative vital force and the Deleuzian concept of *becoming* – oriented toward processes and intensities rather than fixed essences – form the foundation of this perspective. In this way, the categorical distinction between *bios* (human life) and *zoe* (the life of all living beings, including dehumanized humans and non-human animals) is broken down.

Such an approach challenges the Eurocentric gaze of a humanism founded on the binary logic of identity and alterity, where difference becomes the source of hierarchies, exclusions, and essentialisms that degrade those considered "others." Braidotti (2006/2009, p. 70) has mapped these modes of exclusion in a cartography that locates bodies naturalized by humanism and anthropocentrism: the sexualized bodies of women, the racialized bodies of ethnic or Indigenous others, and the non-human bodies of animals and the "others of the earth."

The posthumanist proposal seeks to overcome this legacy through a new conception of subjectivity – one based on the recognition of heterogeneous, hybrid, and multiple coexistences, assembled from their embodied and affective dimension, in constant relation to their surroundings. It is, therefore, an ethical and political stance that embraces diversity, shifting the focus from a unitary subjectivity to a nomadic one. This proposal envisions an expanded notion of community, in which the human is inscribed within a nature–culture continuum that includes all living beings and even the inanimate – technology included.

Technologies, as extensions of human creative capacity, have configured new forms of sensibility and understanding of the environment. From prosthetics that enhance sensory capacities to novel experiences of space and time, these transformations shape what Paula Sibilia (2009) calls a post-organic era – one traversed by the hybridization of the organic and the technological.

Nonetheless, in the midst of this technological expansion, Braidotti (2006/2009) warns of a schizophrenic double bind: on one hand, the consumerist drive for what is always new; on the other, the rejection of any profound change in the human's position relative to other entities. As she notes:

> Thus, the potentially innovative, deterritorializing impact of new technologies is obstructed and distorted by the gravitational pull of old, established values.
>
> (p. 17)

This tension is visible, for example, in the coexistence of atavistic and extremist beliefs alongside cutting-edge narratives about the world. Likewise, a radical emphasis on technology, when it takes on a delirious drive to surpass all limits of the human – closer to the logic of transhumanism – risks turning into an idealized reconfiguration of humanism. This is a reconfiguration that, in aspiring to perfection, may end up denying embodiment and affectivity – constitutive elements of the human condition.

Despite Braidotti's observations (2006/2009, 2013/2015, 2019/2020) about the negative effects technology may have on contemporary subjectivity, her perspective does not adopt an alarmist tone or normative judgements. On the contrary, her reading is guided by the need to recognize the paradoxes that run through current cultural life. This is also the attitude I take in these pages: to avoid both technophobia and technophilia, and not to idealize the past or impose rigid standards of normality or pathology.

My interest lies in understanding how subjectivities are being configured in a transforming world, what kinds of adaptations are possible in the face of emerging tensions, and what maladjustments or disorientations these changes produce in many individuals. Above all, it is crucial for me to emphasize that we are not simply facing an era of many changes, but a genuine change of era. This is a turning point that implies recognizing the human as a complex assemblage, characterized by multiple interconnections and constant transformation

This recognition demands a form of openness that psychoanalysis should not shy away from.

Chords and Assemblages in the Configuration of Subjectivities

Many questions continue to resonate from the proposals posthumanism invites us to consider – questions I will attempt to articulate with certain notions from psychoanalysis. What follows are just a few chords among the many possible.

The first point I would like to raise is that of the human subject. Echoing in my mind is Agamben's (2010) enigmatic question: "What is man, if he is always the place – and, at the same time, the result – of incessant divisions and caesuras?" Or Timothy Morton's (2017/2019) notion of the traumatic rift between the human and the non-human – primarily the animal – concealed within psychic and social space. Both authors allude to a founding, irreducible fracture that recalls the decentred subject of Freudian psychoanalysis: the subject of the unconscious.

This is a subject who, in the turbulence of life, adapts through a plastic and permeable ego, but one that is inevitably fragile and split. An ego that must negotiate with the id and the superego, and through them, with the body, the drive, its phantasms, culture, and even the history of the species (Freud, 1923/1992). R.D. Laing (1960/1975), in his work *The Divided Self*, had already explored the fate of the subject living within such fractured existence. These are sophisticated readings of the complex dynamics of psychic functioning, marked by internal splits and ruptures – readings we must now re-evaluate in light of insights from other disciplines.

From the social field, Bruno Latour (2008) offers a sharp and stimulating perspective that can enrich our thinking. Far from conceiving the social as a cohesive entity, Latour defines it as a kind of relationship among elements that are not, in themselves, inherently social. These heterogeneous components can be reassembled to configure "the bewildering face of the social" (p. 19). This notion of the social as a peculiar movement of re-association and reconfiguration seems particularly relevant for thinking about the psyche.

I propose, then, imagining the psychic assemblage as a space of crossings and negotiations, where the bodily, the drive-related, the affective, the imaginary, the creative, the cultural, the social, the material, nature, and every kind of experience – regardless of origin – are woven together in the play of the psyche.

Theories such as Latour's and Braidotti's prompt us to turn our gaze outward, to observe the reality we share – with whom and under what conditions – recognizing that all of it forms part of the psychic assemblage. They compel us to attend to contemporary transformations and challenge us to generate new ideas around the psychic subject.

For a long time, our attention focused on the work concerning internal reality, neglecting the multiplicity of crossings that constitute it. Today, that gaze is shifting towards the borders, in search of new understandings in the face of unprecedented phenomena. Edges with the body – transsexualities, trans-subjectivities, techno-bodies, among others. Edges with external reality – new experiences of space and time in the virtual era, displacements between the real and the virtual. Borders with social life – globalization, tribalism, polarization, hyperconnectivity. Borders with objects/things – consumerism, dependency, addictions, planned obsolescence. These are just some of the thresholds and the tensions that traverse them.

Objects Created and Creators of Subjectivity

Within the inherently bidirectional nature of transdisciplinarity, psychoanalysis also has much to contribute to the understanding of certain contemporary complexities. This is especially true in the case of Winnicott's contributions, which can enrich the notion of a nomadic and deterritorialized subject. His ideas about the intermediate area of experience – a space that is neither strictly internal nor external, but transitional – are particularly valuable in this regard.

This is a mobile perspective, in which experience is inscribed within a spatiality and temporality in transit: a "between" that does not refer to a fixed location, but rather to a space barely delineated by relationships and to a process in motion, always oriented towards something. These experiences are inscribed in the psychic subject both through an innate drive for development and creativity and through the indispensable participation of the environment, the mother, or the other who enables that becoming.

Let us recall that the creative potential with which the human being is born – a product of their phylogenetic heritage – is only activated insofar as the environment receiving them allows it. In that inaugural encounter, as Winnicott (1971/1995) states, the infant undergoes a foundational experience: the illusion of having created what they need to survive. First, the breast that feeds them; later, other objects that gradually guide them toward a shared reality with others.

Infantile subjectivity would thus emerge from this creative impulse – because of human inventiveness and the multiple transformations it has produced over time. This suggests that a human being is a being in permanent becoming, not a finished entity. In this way, they do not merely adapt to the world: they also create it. The human subject not only generates their affectively significant objects but also projects that same creative gesture onto multiple objects or things they will come to feel are essential to their existence.

Is it not possible, then, to consider that this creative development, as conceptualized in psychoanalysis, could help us better understand the intense relationship with technological objects highlighted by posthumanist theories? The creative capacity, first configured in the experience of illusion, is projected into that intermediate zone where cultural experience takes place. And within it, virtual phenomena are also inscribed: language, writing, science, technology – everything that continues that unfolding.

We live in amphibian times. We are learning to recognize that we inhabit a liminal dimension in which diverse realities, processes, and substrates are interconnected. Like a polyphony of voices and instruments – body, emotions, senses, creativity, relationships, technical supports, screens, processors, and machines – everything intermingles and fuses into what we perceive as the experience of everyday life. It is a "warp of material, biocultural, and symbolic forces that participate in the formation of the subject," as Braidotti (2006/2009, p. 61) puts it.

Winnicott's valuable notion of the creation of significant objects is not the only one psychoanalysis has to offer. Already in Freud, object cathexis implied that objects acquired psychic value for the subject. Although the Freudian perspective is oriented primarily towards human objects, it is precisely Freud's conceptualization of perversion and the contingency of the object that grants great malleability to the capacity to invest different types of objects affectively.

André Green (1995/1996), for his part, expands this line of thought by developing the idea of an *objectalizing function*, which – in tension with a *de-objectalizing drive* – accounts for the vicissitudes of the life and death drives. These forces are manifested in the bond – and its rupture – with created objects, expressing the structural oscillations of the psyche between connection and disconnection.

In any of these psychoanalytic approaches, objects or things gain relevance from the subject's perspective – that is, from the human capacity for invention. The bonds established with these objects can extend to other human beings, animals, or even inanimate objects, as long as they retain psychic value for the subject.

These objects – inanimate but "animated" in their psychic function – can fulfil various roles: companions, attachment figures, transitional objects, addictive objects, fetishes, and more. All of them illustrate how, according to psychoanalytic theories, the external can be subjectively invested and become part of the subject's affective fabric.

The philosopher Roberto Esposito (2017) aims to dismantle the rigid historical division between persons and things. He notes, however, that in some primitive societies, this relationship was conceived through a logic of complementarity: a more vital connection with the inanimate, akin to an animistic experience that promoted respect for the life of things.

Esposito argues that only by stepping outside the opposition between person and thing and situating ourselves in an intermediate terrain can we perceive the complexity of the bond that unites them. In this sense, he presents the body as the site where things interact with human beings to the point of becoming a kind of symbolic and material extension of them (Esposito, 2017, p. 26).

What happens, then, with objects that become part of the body – transplants, implants, and prostheses? How should we understand the growing universe of objects endowed with artificial intelligence that interact at multiple levels of individual and social life, inevitably affecting the psychic assemblage? These objects, though increasingly naturalized, are still scarcely addressed by psychoanalysis. Posthumanist theories have decisively addressed these questions. Braidotti (2006/2009, 2013/2015, 2019/2020), for example, proposes that the interdependence between bodies and technology gives rise to a new symbiotic relationship. Within this framework, cybernetic organisms or technobodies are constituted as the subjects of our contemporary culture, immersed in a complex network of social dynamics mediated by technology.

From Esposito's (2017) perspective, these technobodies should not be objects of nostalgia or perceived as threats, but rather recognized as another expression of the technological animal we have always been. This idea is also supported by Maureira (2016), who claims that we have always been cyborgs, alluding to our constitutive relationship with technology since the very origins of humanity.

This is especially true if we understand technology as the Greeks did, under the notion of *téchne*: that which is produced by human intelligence and over which some degree of control is – or is believed to be – exercised.

Following this trajectory, it becomes essential to critically examine the relationship between subjectivation processes – always mobile and in flux – and the vast and mutable unfolding of technological creation. This involves attempting a reflection from psychoanalysis that does not limit itself to considering technology's impact on the psyche, but rather starts from the recognition of the technobody and the ways in which it is psychically represented.

Hybridization or the Colonialism of the Algorithm

In an attempt to think through philosophy, psychoanalysis, neurology, and the cognitive sciences, Benasayag and Pennisi (2023) argue that we are facing a contemporary issue marked by the colonization of the algorithm. This algorithm promotes a life reduced to points and precisions, rather than lines, processes, or segments, concealing a positivism that presents itself as neutral and devoid of ideology. Yet, its logic ultimately serves a supposedly greater good: productive efficiency governed by the logic of capital.

What gets displaced in this perspective is life itself – its complexity, imperfections, nuances, variability, and the multiplicity of its singularities. A deep tension is thus established between the One – the homogeneous, systematized by global macroeconomics – and the Multiple, which insists on resisting. This multiplicity is expressed not only in cultural differences but also in bodily experience, which is always situated, embodied, and context-specific, even as it becomes increasingly deterritorialized.

This "algorithmic colonialism" imposes a matrix of the One that induces subjects to identify with alien forms of existence, generating deep alienation. People become captured by these algorithmic spaces – always imaginary – which eliminate room for difference, singular experience, and the symbolic.

Benasayag, in Benasayag and Pennisi (2023), warns that although hybridization is part of natural evolution – especially human evolution – when alterity is ignored, such hybridization becomes a colonizing gesture. It is not only about the relationship between humans and technology (or between different cultures) but also about acknowledging the existence of differentiated entities participating in the encounter. When technology does not coexist with alterity, but instead subsumes it, what arises is no longer hybridization, but a mimetic project: the attempt to adapt the living to the ideal of the machine, eliminating everything deemed defective or inefficient in the human. In that gesture, the possibility of mutual transformation disappears, giving way to a form of domination – a new colonialism that erases difference under the promise of technical perfection.

With this problematization of the situation in mind, how then are we to conceptualize the hybridization between the technobody and the libidinal body? What can be said about its symbolic inscription? These questions open a fertile ground for exploring new forms of subjectivity in a time marked by increasingly complex assemblages of the organic, the psychic, the social, and the technical.

Braidotti (2006/2009) proposes a cultural figure that infuses bodily experience and may well extend to libidinal experience. While she does not claim to offer a definitive explanation of the evolution of identities and gender relations, her position is strikingly provocative. She argues that, unlike in earlier eras when the machinic double of the body was heavily sexualized – as in the phallic figures of steam or locomotives – postmodernity has introduced an electronic and digital machinery composed of

> figures of complexity, mixture, hybridity, and interconnection. As such, they are not associated with gender nor particularly sexualized; rather, they mark a space of indeterminacy, an undecidable space of transsexuality.
>
> (Braidotti, 2006/2009, p. 77)

Thus, she links the silent impact of technological development to the progressive dissolution of the boundaries of sexual difference, guiding the contemporary subject toward a kind of generalized androgyny. The disembodiment and anonymity that accompany virtual experience may have also contributed in that direction.

It is worth recalling that, for psychoanalysis, psychosexuality encompasses not only drive, body, desire, fantasy, emotions, and relationships, but also history, culture, and therefore, gender.

It is becoming less controversial to establish a legitimate conceptual relationship between the psychoanalytic understanding of sexuality and gender theories. Nonetheless, this convergence has not been without resistance – likely rooted in the weight of biology and the lingering effects of a dichotomous mode of thought still present in many knowledge domains.

This is the same pendular logic that has led psychoanalysis into sterile debates, such as the opposition between the primacy of the drive or the object, or the false dichotomy between intrapsychic and intersubjective psychoanalysis. These theoretical fractures, which narrow our ability to grasp complexity, are akin to the clinical rigidity often associated with pathology: the fixedness that prevents movement.

Therefore, I agree with Braidotti (2009, 2013, 2020) on the need to rethink the affects promoted by technoculture from a more neutral perspective – that is, without pathologizing what we do not yet understand merely to force reality into our theoretical frameworks. This attitude is particularly crucial in addressing the forms of discomfort emerging around new experiences of sexuality, eroticism, and gender, as well as in relation to processes of technological hybridization.

As humans, we interpret reality through certain perceptive faculties – visual, auditory – along with cerebral processes and accumulated narratives. While we think of ourselves as primarily rational beings, we are, in essence, survival machines: creative, yes, but fundamentally transformers of information. We are apparatuses of reverie, in the Bionian sense (Bion, 1967/1977), attempting to metabolize and give symbolic form to every experience – both our own and that of others.

But this capacity requires a gradual learning process, and even then, it remains a deeply imperfect and arduous task. When we add to this the constant transformation of the environment and of ourselves, it becomes understandable that difficulties and maladaptations arise – or at least significant delays in achieving adaptation. Considering the speed imposed by digital tempo, we can see serious obstacles to subjective elaboration and the availability of spaces for experience.

Furthermore, if we acknowledge the existence of subjective multiplicities, it would be a mistake to continue upholding a narrow range of ways of being as the "healthy norm." It is essential not to lose sight of our commitment to listening to the unconscious, understanding the desiring subject, and expanding their symbolic capacity. But we must also remember that psychoanalysis is more than a psychology: its perspective on complexity subverts any normative parameter aligned with a fixed health canon, and should therefore remain open to exploring the evolving forms of eroticism and their articulation within gender and power relations.

Coda: Polyphony as a Figure of Contemporary Thought

A guiding question for this conclusion is how to articulate the singularity of the psychoanalytic subject with the notion of a relational and transhuman subject proposed by posthumanist epistemologies. Can psychoanalysis, with its emphasis on the particular, engage in dialogue with these amplified configurations of being? How can we integrate multiple forms of existence without diluting the attentive listening to singularity that defines the analytic experience?

In an attempt to shed light on some of these questions, I have felt inclined to turn to the field of music and use polyphony not only as a metaphor but also as a model. It seems particularly fruitful to think about the human condition through the notion of an entanglement of heterogeneous multiplicities within a system that, although seemingly homogeneous and ordered, preserves singular voices and is capable of tolerating the chaos of dissonance, atonality, and cacophony.

Polyphony offers us a complex figure of what is simultaneously singular and diverse, without one dimension annulling the other. In music, polyphony embraces the momentum without losing the continuity of the process, replicating the very origin of musicality in the vibration that runs through all living matter – and even the inanimate – as Reich (1984/2008) suggests. Everything in nature, for biological or physical reasons, vibrates in multiple and diverse tempos. Each entity has its own rhythm, a singular temporality, but resonates with the rhythms of everything else in a polyphonic manner.

Throughout the history of polyphony, we can also discern an analogous tension: that between the humanist ideal of ordered perfection – evident in canonical academic European polyphony later extended across the West – and a broader evolutionary vision, whose origin may lie in the collective, dissonant, and seemingly chaotic singing of early hominids, meant to generate shared protection in the face of threat. It is this latter perspective I wish to highlight, for it has evolved into musicality in multiple cultural expressions, particularly in the traditions of Oceania, Asia, and Africa, creating increasingly complex networks of social interdependence since the beginnings of humanity.

A key concept that reinforces this choice is transposition, which Braidotti (2006/2009) borrows from both music and genetics to describe movements within a discontinuous but harmonious framework. She defines it as

> an intertextual transfer that traverses borders transversally, in the sense of moving from one code, field, or axis to another. . . , not in the sense of plural multiplication but of complex multiplicities.
>
> (Braidotti, 2006/2009, p. 20)

Beyond its emphasis on complex multiplicities, what particularly interests me about this notion is the possibility of transposing concepts across disciplines – of allowing thought to circulate and expand in new directions. Hence my interest in embracing the posthumanist challenge through a polyphonic transdisciplinarity, which is essential for approaching the complexity of contemporary subjectivities.

I would like to close these reflections – closer to a *work in progress* than to a finished argument – with a quote from Étienne Souriau (1943/2017), which beautifully condenses what I have sought to express throughout this text:

> Everything – ourselves, a rock, a bird, a table, an atom – is unfinished, halfway there, as if given in half-light. Every act of existing demands effort, a process, and therefore, an art. There are no subjects or objects, rather combinations yet to be made, emerging through echoes and mutual responses . . . a plurality of fragmentary and inherently arbitrary voices that sometimes produce a chord.
>
> (p. 66)

References

Agamben, G. (2010). *Lo abierto. El hombre y el animal*. Pre-Textos.

Benasayag, M., & Pennisi, A. (2023). *La inteligencia artificial no piensa (El cerebro tampoco)*: Prometeo Editorial.

Bion, W. (1977). *Volviendo a pensar*. Paidos. (Original work published 1967)

Braidotti, R. (2009). *Transposiciones*. Editorial Gedisa. (Original work published 2006)

Braidotti, R. (2015). *Lo posthumano*. Editorial Gedisa. (Original work published 2013)

Braidotti, R. (2020). *El conocimiento posthumano*. Editorial Gedisa. (Original work published 2019)

Espósito, R. (2017). *Personas, cuerpos, cosas*. Editorial Trotta.

Freud, S. (1997). El Yo y el Ello. In *Obras completas*, Vol. XIX. Amorrortu. (Original work published 1923)

Green, A. (1996). *La metapsicología revisitada*. Eudeba. (Original work published 1995)

Jullien, F. (2013). *Cinco conceptos propuestos al psicoanálisis*. El cuenco de plata.

Laing, R. (1975). *El yo dividido*. Fondo de cultura económica. (Original work published 1960)

Latour, B. (2008). *Reensamblar lo social. Una introducción a la teoría del actor-red*. Manantial.

Maureira, M. (2016). Posthumanismo: más allá de antropotécnica y nomadismo. *Cinta Moebio*, *55*, 1–15. www.moebio.uchile.cl/55/maureira.html

Morin, E. (2011). *Introducción al pensamiento complejo*. Gedisa. (Original work published 1990)

Morton, T. (2019). *Humanidad. Solidaridad con los no-humanos*. Adriana Hidalgo editora. (Original work published 2017)

Nosek, L. (2017). *A disposição para o assombro*. Perspectiva.

Puget, J. (2020). Vivir e desequilibrio permanente. *Fronteras*. Libro Virtual del 33 Congreso Latinoamericano de Psicoanálisis. http://montevideo2020.fepal.org/

Reich, S. (2008). Music as a gradual process. In P. Weiss & R. Taruskin (Eds.), *Music in the western world*. Thomson Learning Academic. (Original work published 1984)

Sibilia, P. (2013). *El hombre post-orgánico: cuerpo, subjetividad y tecbologías digitales*. Fondo de Cultura económica. (Original work published 2009)

Souriau, É. (2017). Del modo de existencia de la obra por hacer. In Isabelle Stengers and Bruno Latour (eds), *Los diferentes modos de existencia*. Cactus. (Original work published 1943)

Winnicott, D. (1995). *Realidad y juego*. Editorial Gedisa. (Original work published 1971)

11 The Flesh, the Last Bastion of the Colonizable

Helga Fernández

Translated by Carolina Glaser[1]

I

From gymnastics and sport in Greco-Roman Antiquity, through the asceticism of the cilice, monastic abstinence, the knightly nobility of the Middle Ages, the desecration of tombs and dissection of corpses during the Renaissance, to the prevalence of the face and the gaze in modernity, and finally to contemporary times with its technomorphisms, the body is conceived and treated through various ethics and aesthetics. However, if history is written from the perspective of the victors, it must also be acknowledged that, over the course of time, the body has been stripped of its entrails, its semen, its tears, its saliva, its laughter, its joys, and its miseries. In order to avoid disregarding embodiment and giving substance to the current era, it is crucial to recognize that the asepsis of history is sustained by dualism. Whether understood as the dichotomy between extended substance and thinking substance, or between body and mind, dualism produces a tension that subjects the body to two opposing poles: denigration or idealization. If denigrated, the body is perceived as obscene and concupiscent, leading to its rejection; if idealized, it is sacralized and abstracted, resulting in its avoidance.

In Descartes' philosophy (1641/2009), the point of junction between soul and body is a mystery, while remaining beyond doubt. The Sixth Meditation is devoted to this issue, and within its paragraphs a third substance is mentioned – between the thinking and the extended. A substance which, unlike bodies and ideas, can only be felt, but neither thought nor represented. Several years later, Husserl (1952/1997) identifies this (substance?) as flesh, *meinen Leib*, and explicitly distinguishes it from the body. This is the same flesh taken up by Merleau-Ponty (1964/2010) in *The Visible and the Invisible*, a work that in turn becomes the thread with which Lacan (2006) weaves the *objet* a as a pound of flesh.

In its translation – from Hebrew (*basar*) to Greek (σάρξ, σαρκός) and Latin (*caro, carnis*) – flesh is the site of an incommensurability between two opposing instances: body (σῶμα) and soul (ψυχή), body and spirit (πνεῦμα, breath, air, spirit). Flesh inaugurates an insurmountable interval that separates both

DOI: 10.4324/9781003783862-16

terms, thus requiring a ternary rhetoric that challenges dualisms while being unable to dispense with them. As a third instance, flesh disrupts the soul/body dualism and offers the opportunity to refute a position that opposes the desiring body to a *Logos* which, having been insidiously and surreptitiously disembodied, appears pallid and impalpable. At the same time, it allows us to resist reducing the body to a *jouissance*, which – having been perfidiously and clandestinely severed from the Word – presents itself solely as vice and excess.

II

In our present moment, a series of events – whose common denominator is a particular way of engaging with the most visceral aspects of the body – has been unfolding. Given that these events challenge, redefine, and in some cases aim to transcend the impossible – as a gesture toward opening the horizon explored in this work – I propose to read them according to the following formulation: The forclusion[2] of flesh from the Real, returning through its imaginary consistency (a conjecture I attempt to cipher and decipher throughout the course of this journey).

Some Events

1. Some time ago, two movements emerged on the world stage: Russian Cosmism and universal Transhumanism (Bana & Galliano, 2021).

   The abolition of time and space were the two central proposals of the action programme that, at the turn of the 19th to the 20th century, brought together a group of Russian authors, novelists, radical anarchists, revolutionary activists, poets, philosophers, scientists, and pioneers of astronautics. According to cosmism principles, human beings should overcome their differences and unite their efforts toward this common goal, which would be followed by interplanetary conquest. While in Russia this endeavour sought to advance its objective through technology, Julian Huxley – Aldous's brother – in Great Britain, proposed:

   > The human species can, if it wishes, transcend itself – not just sporadically, an individual here in one way, an individual there in another way – but in its entirety, as humanity. We need a name for this new belief. Perhaps transhumanism will serve: man remaining man, but transcending himself.
   >
   > (Huxley, 1957, p. 13)

   Under the concept of transhumanism, Huxley developed a line of thought that, similar to the co-epochal movement in Russia, is grounded in a Darwinian-style anti-naturalism. As part of the very process of the humanity's unlimited modification, it conceives the human being as a plastic device capable of transformation through physical processes.

Over time, both movements entered a phase of latency, only to reawaken in the late 1980s. In 1988, Max More, influenced by the body-freezing pioneer Robert Ettinger, revived the project by founding a new movement – Extropy – led by white men who were antifeminist, anti-environmentalist, libertarian, and sympathetic to racism. Today, the main proposals of Cosmism and Transhumanism – in some ways fused – are carried out by Silicon Valley ventures such as Google's California Life Company or experiments funded by Peter Thiel, PayPal's co-founder, all of which renew the quest for immortality through advances in a language detached from the flesh.

2. Eugenia Kuyda, co-founder of LUKA (an artificial intelligence platform), was inspired by an episode of the series *Black Mirror*, "Be Right Back" (Harris, 2013 (Web Articles/News Media)), to programme a bot that mimics the speech patterns of a deceased loved one (*El Español*, 2023). Friends and family supported the project and provided their digital conversations with Roman Mazurenko so they could be processed. Sometime later, the existence of the bot was announced, stating that anyone who downloaded the app could talk to him, in both Russian and English, by messaging the user @Roman. "Roman, this is your digital monument" – wrote Eugenia.

   Other close ones who disagreed with the project stated: "Roman needs a memorial, but not like this."

   "This isn't virtual reality – it's a new reality, and we have to get used to it," the programmer replied.
3. In Taiwan, it has been reported that some people, after playing for 3, 4, 7 days, or more without stopping – not even to use the bathroom or eat – die. This phenomenon is called "gaming death" (Parkin, 2021).
4. There are interactive smart vibrators and male masturbators that allow the exact movements of a video to be synchronized with the penis. There are also pillows capable of reproducing a heartbeat, and a gadget that brings the kiss of someone who might be on the other side of the world to our lips, through force sensors.
5. In the terms and conditions of the Amazon Web Services guide, clause 42.10 states that the Lumberyard materials – the free 3D game engine – were not designed for use in life-critical or safety-critical systems, unless humans suffer an infection that turns them into zombies (*El Diario.es*, 2023). The clause reads as follows:

   > The Lumberyard materials are not intended for use with life-critical or safety-critical systems, such as use in operation of medical equipment, automated transportation systems, autonomous vehicles, aircraft or air traffic control, nuclear facilities, manned spacecraft, or military use in connection with live combat. However, this restriction will not apply in the event . . . of a widespread viral infection transmitted via bites or contact with bodily fluids that causes human corpses to reanimate and seek to consume living human flesh, blood, brain, or nerve tissue, and is likely to result in the fall of organized civilization.

6. When the pandemic began, in some football stadiums, fans were replaced by dolls or robots (*Ciudad Magazine*, 2020). These dolls are also sold in separate parts to assemble the "ideal woman" to suit those gentlemen who find pleasure in their daily company, and used in brothels to provide sexual services to clients. An engineer from one of the factories behind these prototypes stated that approaching them is like surrounding the heart with mirrors, and that one needs something to love, because no being can become human without contact with an object of love – even if that object is a doll (Greiner, 2019).
7. The Cybernetic Culture Research Unit (CCRU) was founded in 1995 within the Department of Philosophy at the University of Warwick, initially under the direction of Sadie Plant and shortly thereafter under Nick Land. The group continued operating semi-clandestinely until 2003. During that time, among other pursuits, it focused on the artificial creation of realities, referred to as hyperstitional.

   Hyperstition (CCRU, 2022) is a semiotic production liberated from speaking beings which brings itself into reality. A paradigmatic example of digital hyperstition is the case of Slenderman – an entity that originated as creepypasta[3] on internet forums and became real the moment two 12-year-old girls from the US state of Wisconsin stabbed a classmate 19 times in an attempt to kill her, in 2014. When asked what had motivated the act, they testified that Slenderman had appeared to them, claiming that if they wanted to live in his mansion in the woods and become his servants, they had to kill that person. Hyperstition often emerges through horror – as in this case, where the actions of the two girls ultimately transformed a plausible object into a verifiable one. Yet there are countless examples of how, through human sacrifice, synthetic truth enters the material world of flesh-and-blood bodies.

The Performativity of the Flesh

From the 19th century onwards, it seems necessary to admit that certain technological advances have enabled ideologies to capture a dimension of the body, thereby blurring the boundary between the human and the artificial; they "overcome" limitations, provoke sexual arousal through electrical stimulation, simulate deceased loved ones to continue speaking and writing, allow humans to be replaced by dolls, and create synthetic realities that dispense with consensus and legitimacy grounded in the interwoven structure of society.

However, despite all attempts and achievements of domestication, subjugation, and transformation, one dimension of the body also constitutes the materialization of a space of resistance and revolt against such policies. Thus, although this force of rejection operates within the finitude of the human body – sometimes to the extreme of a genuine will to annihilation justified by its "defects" – something excessive, marginalized, unsymbolizable returns in the form of threat, obscenity, and contagion, as if an irreducible presence manifests itself before the very discourse that expels it from itself: the flesh.

Through its raw presence or its blazing absence, flesh holds a preeminent place in our time. It is invoked in street posters advocating veganism. It is sold as an artificial product. It is piled up at borders, through the desecration of the bodies of those fleeing their homelands. It inspires dystopias and fuels essays. It becomes a limit to be eradicated in scientific projects that pursue immortality.

Emerging from an imaginary of dangerous, degenerate carnality – manifesting as scientific-sounding delusional ideas (such as Amazon's contract) or through film, series, fiction, and visual arts – it becomes manifest that what has been expelled returns in terrifying forms. The forclusion of flesh returns in inanimate objects that colonize the place of the Other, in monstrous, formless, and threatening crowds, and in devices that seem to re-establish the rejected affect through a kind of technological hypersensitivity.

Flesh, in its irreducibility, reveals itself as a reminder of our helplessness (Hilflosigkeit), resisting the attempts of dematerialization and abstraction of the digital era. Despite technological and scientific advances that aim to exclude and transcend it, flesh persists as the site where sexuality and death are inscribed. In its wounds and lacerations, in its Real presentation and imaginary consistency, flesh exposes what it had kept secret beneath the skin: the nakedness of its untamed materiality. Torn, it becomes the surface on which the domination and cruelty of an ethics/aesthetics are written – reducing it to just another thing among things; or it incites speech and thereby the survival of another ethics/aesthetics: that of the subject of the unconscious.

Flesh enacts its performativity.

Body and Flesh

If the Symbolic tends toward incorporation and produces corporealities sustained by diverse supports, the only thing that attests to a body being human is mental weakness (Lacan, 1974–1975) and the incarnated word.

But flesh is not the body; it is what a body is not. For a body to differentiate itself from flesh, something must be lost – and from that loss emerges the cause of a sentient body, not merely a sensed one; a body that gives, not only is given; that speaks, not only is spoken. A body that makes itself felt, makes itself offered, makes itself heard – at the other extreme of auto-eroticism (Henry, 2001). Flesh and body are constituted through a certain bond, although, at times, this bond implies that the body fails to cover the flesh. Flesh bears inscribed the body of the Symbolic,[4] which makes the body naive. The Symbolic does not reach to touch the most Real of life. The Real is also reflected by the Imaginary, giving rise to a representation of the body that aligns with mental weakness. The body we have is an effect of the body of the Symbolic. Flesh forms part of the soma, but it does not fully commune with it; something in flesh often serves as the surface for the inscription of the Other.

But when the mark is not possible, flesh is impressed – to the paroxysm of the stigma, or to the numbness of indifference. The body can change body, ideal, and conception; it can be thought, created, and legislated by culture. Flesh, although partially touched and processed by language, remains the last redoubt of the colonizable. The body reaches a level of abstraction. Flesh is where sex and death happen. The body aspires to a certain sophistication and empowerment. Flesh confronts us with the limit and the literalness of the impossible. The body aspires to immortality and lays claim to the eternal. Flesh is the evidence that life, in its raw state, leads to annihilation. The body is an effect of representations. Flesh does not represent: it underpins all metaphor, but cannot be metaphorized. Flesh is flesh.

The Flesh in Question

No language suffices for flesh. What remains to encode it then is either the excess of minimalism or the extravagance of ornamentation. But the matter is not simple – we are faced with two conditions that hinder the task: its forgetting and its presentification.

1. If flesh gives body to metaphor, it becomes veiled and repressed – clothed in the Signifier or adorned with words – while simultaneously emerging as representation and figuration. It also stands as evidence of what the Symbolic dimension cannot grasp: that is, as both limit and object a.
2. If flesh does not give body to metaphor, nor becomes embodied within it, it emerges in the place of das Ding – in a dismembered or fragmented body, in the Real stumps of hallucination, and in the stigma. It also appears as an effect of the passion of the Signifier, when the unary trait fails and there is a drive toward restitution through literal marks that wound the surface of a skin opening into flesh, and, in its maximal consistency, in the return within the imaginary after its forclusion from the real.

The designation "flesh" does not refer to *res extensa* nor to the organism; it points to the Symbolic–Imaginary confirmation of a Real in which language either anchors or fails to anchor. It is the naming of a material substratum without which the mirror-stage body, the body of subject identification, and the erogenous body would not exist. It refers to the "mystery of the speaking body" (Lacan, 1972–1973/2012a), to that ground where the Signifier anchors and produces affect. Flesh does not fully coincide with what we call the real body, which Lacan names, in the Borromean knot, life (Lacan, 1975): it may be located in the advance of the mortification of the symbolic dimension within the real.

Throughout this exploration, flesh is not conceived as the biological foundation of a fixed fate; rather, it is considered an element which, like earth, air, fire, and water, possesses its own qualities. Flesh carries within itself its own decay and perishability – it confronts us with the not-possible and the impossible. The composition and decomposition of its vibrant matter reveal that we are made of the same substance as algae, elephants, meteorites, and birch trees: a shared materiality that reorients any anthropocentric perspective, while also reminding us that humans inhabit their own specificity.

Human flesh bears two properties that either oppose or intertwine: its refractoriness to the Symbolic, and its elasticity within the Signifier. The first is expressed in the literalness through which every metaphor is absorbed and erased; the second becomes evident in the body's ductility and agility, in its transmutation by language into the invisible and incorporeal. When both properties underpin one another, flesh does not hinder metaphor, nor does language drive toward an annihilating omnipotence. Flesh cushions the drift of the Signifier, sets limits to the sumptuousness of the Symbolic, and constitutes the fabric of speech, just as language abandons its machinic cadence and softens its rhetorical excess. Despite its refractoriness to the Symbolic – and precisely because of this – flesh is the site from which metaphor originates, the zero point of all ciphering, and the locus where every signification – literal or metaphorical, achieved or failed – interlocks. Every weave of words is umbilically tied to the flesh. All language is "organ language."

We are speaking beings constituted between two second natures: one of language, the other of flesh. Word and flesh intermingle, such that in the *parlêtre* the process of incarnation takes place – not only as mythic but also as structural. Yet, once the mythical or logical origin has occurred, flesh is already human flesh: *chair*, not *viande*. Just as the speaking being may stand outside the word but not outside language, neither can they inhabit a flesh without marks. And even as the flesh is further altered by the Symbolic – through the instillation of the Signifier – it does so according to its own singularities. There will thus be a modality of flesh in which this transformative process takes hold, and another in which the Signifier fails to fully take root.

In the immixtion[5] of the Symbolic/Real of the Word with the Real of flesh, the latter is animated, cadaverized, and the Word itself is vivified. Or, when the Word becomes flesh, it reveals itself as symbolically Symbolic, emerging from a Symbolic/Real; just as when it becomes entangled in the flesh, the flesh emerges as a Real/Symbolic. As with the entanglement of the life and death drives, it becomes necessary to consider a link between flesh and Word – so that the Word does not besiege the speaking being as command or schizophrenic abstraction, and so that flesh does not literalize the subtlety of the Signifier to the point of erasing all difference.

Flesh and Word, when split, propel toward some form of excess. To expect everything from the servility of language – reducing it to a mere instrument – and to reject flesh as that which also inscribes us result in an anaesthesia of what affects, and an impotence, or disempowerment, of that which affects. To expect everything from flesh – reducing it to a surface of jouissance – and to reject language as that which also constitutes us lead beyond the pleasure principle and into an ever-deepening silence. Flesh is altered by the Symbolic, and the Symbolic expresses – or reveals – itself in profoundly different ways when it is incorporated into flesh, as opposed to when it is taken up by a létouse.[6] Likewise, when it is transmitted from one fleshy body to another, or from a metallic body to one of flesh.

III

From the way each discourse – political, religious, scientific, transhumanist, posthumanist, psychoanalytic, capitalist, technocratic, culinary, artistic, social, and so on – acts upon flesh, different ethics/aesthetics are produced. In the case of this work, there are three ethics/aesthetics: the one enacted by psychoanalysis, beginning with the dream of Irma's injection; the one driven by science in its alliance with cybernetics, through the forclusion of flesh; and finally, the one composed by the art of David Cronenberg.

Irma's Injection Dream: Flesh as the Threshold of the Unconscious

The place where Lacan most closely refers to flesh in the sense invoked here is in his paraphrasing of the dream of Irma's injection:

> There is a horrible discovery here: the flesh that is never seen, the foundation of things, the reverse of the face, of the visage, the secrets *par excellence*, the flesh from which everything emerges, at the very heart of mystery, the suffering, formless flesh, whose very shape provokes anxiety. Vision of anxiety, identification of anxiety, the last revelation of **you are this**: You are this, which is the farthest from you, the most formless.
>
> (Lacan, 1954–1955/1993, pp. 235–236)

Freud dreams the inaugural dream of psychoanalysis as a nightmare from which, nonetheless, he does not wake up. What allows him to resolve the identification of anxiety is that, from the infected pustules, the formula of trimethylamine emerges: the cipher of the solution of the word, in bold strokes (Freud, 1900/1979). A cipher is the product of the action of the Symbolic which, as a treatment of the literalness of flesh, immixes with it; it is also the mortification of the Signifier entering into the Real of life; and furthermore, it is the intrusion of language, which, within the materiality of a certain dimension of the body, is branded as letter. Trimethylamine is a product of the decomposition of animals and plants – the substance responsible for the smell of rotten fish, infections, and bad breath. At this point, we decompose, there are no longer bodies; flesh degrades and fuses with the earth.

In his inaugural dream, the structure unfolds toward its complexity. Freud does not leap out of bed in horror at the grotesque vision, because the ethical position that inhabits him, and the desire that guides him, render the putrefied flesh a fallow ground for the Symbolic. The dream's progression traces a passage from the Imaginary to the formlessness of flesh, and from there to the literal inoculation – the infection of language as a gateway to the unconscious.

Even if the Real may awaken, there is no exit from where pustules ferment unless the wedge is touched – the Real anchor of the Word: flesh. The same flesh from which life emerges. The same flesh that can devour with its necrotizing darkness. The same flesh that, consequently, is the wall on which every difference is inscribed or absorbed.

The dream of the injection shuts the jaws of flesh by opening the speaking mouth. Flesh is immixed by the Symbolic and, as an effect, is veiled by the skin. It exits the Real that regresses toward destruction and touches the Real that is navelled to the Symbolic. The inaugural dream reveals that flesh becomes visceral when it is made so – when it is viscerally engaged or wounded – or becomes the support of speech when it is infected and affected by an ethics/aesthetics caused by the imperative: "Let it be said!"

The Forclusion of Flesh

In Lacan's teaching, at least six forms of forclusion (*Verwerfung*) can be identified: *Verwerfung* of the feminine (Lacan, 1957–1958/1999), *Verwerfung* of the phallus (1958), *Verwerfung* of the subject's being (1958), Verwerfung of love in the capitalist discourse (1972), *Verwerfung* of the commandments of speech (1975), and *Verwerfung* of meaning (1976). In 1960, Lacan also asserts that science performs a Verwerfung of the Thing and, later, a *Verwerfung* of truth as cause. Furthermore, regarding capitalist discourse, in 1972 he argues that it enacts a *Verwerfung* of castration. This series of nominations appears to seek the specificity of this forceful rejection and to trace its mutations, as they relate to the singularities of each historical moment.

I propose to read the *Verwerfung* of flesh as belonging to the same order as other forms of forclusion operating in this epoch, but with particularities that stem from its alliance with cybernetics as an ideology that enacts a praxis upon the body. Perhaps it is the specific forclusion of our epochality, through which an inescapable dimension of the body is expelled. Not the Imaginary body, nor the Symbolic body, but the living body. That body which touches and is touched.

The forclusion of flesh is operated by science and technology, but it can also manifest in the speaking being and in the discourse of psychoanalysis. This occurs particularly when the latter asserts that the body in question is not the body of flesh and bone, thereby forcluding the material substrate upon which all dimensions of the body are grounded. This forclusion takes place when only the distance and ectopia of the pulsional body, the virtual presentation of the specular body, and the metamorphoses of the Symbolic body are considered – as if these latter existed prior to and beyond the flesh, or even freed from it.

To consider forclusion as a mode of exclusion so forceful that what is excluded returns in a different dimension from the one it was rejected from, is a way to approach the treatment of forclusions both in the parlêtre and in the structure of discourses. At the same time, it allows us to distinguish that the forclusion of the Name-of-the-Father enacts a suppression in the Symbolic dimension (Lacan, 1955–1956), while the forclusion of flesh operates as a rejection of the Real. This is why, in the forclusion of the Name-of-the-Father, what is excluded from the Symbolic returns in the Real, whereas, in the forclusion of the living body, what is excluded from the Real[7] returns in the Imaginary – at its most condensed, as the opposite of the incorporeal: a coagulated or compact substance.

Every Imaginary has substance, and this is what gives it consistency by reflecting the Real, by doubling it (Lacan, 1974–1975/1993). The more forcefully the Real of the flesh is forcluded, the more it returns in less elastic forms – ones even more literal than its own irreducibility. The forclusion of the Real produces, as an effect, presentifications that are not representations, but appearances of what ought to exist through ex-sistence: unburied corpses, zombies, tin dolls colonizing the space of the Other, and souls packaged into chips . . .

Cybernetics, as an ideology that enacts a praxis upon the body, is the framework and discipline that most clearly reveals the forclusion of the flesh, insofar as it tends toward a dematerialization nourished by a dystopian ideal: one in which eternity would be achieved through the refinement of algorithms capable of abstracting and storing the soul – made possible by the existence of the Symbolic body and the specular body, as well as by the literalization of the immortality of flesh, conceived as a progress yet to be conquered.

A New Flesh?

The dissection, the brutal treatment, and the eroticism of flesh in the film *Crimes of the Future* (David Cronenberg, 2022) could resemble a staging from the late Middle Ages or the early Renaissance, when the dissection of corpses was a common practice carried out by anatomists who wrote treatises in verse and by painters who studied the geography of cadavers to create their works. Cronenberg's aesthetic composes the image by juxtaposing living flesh with rusted metals – something that could not have occurred during the Renaissance. In *Crimes of the Future*, the tins belong to an old, abandoned, obsolete, and apparently delibidinized world, which nonetheless continues to sustain cameras, televisions, and other gadgets.

These devices, moreover, seem to continue to inscribe the human, camouflaged. Remote controls, for instance, perceive[8] the body's physiology and possess a materiality similar to flesh, as if they had taken its image and replicated it. The protagonist, Saul Tenser, sleeps in an organic cradle connected to his body by tentacles that anticipate pain and reposition him to sleep. None of these biomechanical objects bear any trace of tin in their components: there are no chips, silicon, or screens. Everything appears made of flesh and bone, skin, mucosa, and scab.

When flesh is forcluded – in its suffering and perishability – it returns through its consistency from within the Imaginary, demanding a form of jouissance once science has stripped it of the one it formerly practised. In the Cronenbergian habitat, where pain and pleasure have perished, new forms of jouissance are invented: cuts, amputations, and surgeries. "Surgery is the new sex," declares an instituting official. "The body is reality," is displayed on screens no one seems to watch. What has been extinguished is not the létouses nor the ideology techniques, but the veiling of flesh and skin as mask and shelter – and thus, representation, and nearly metaphor itself. There is no other canvas but the body itself, dissected: flesh. There, the brushstroke is the instrument that marks and wounds the entrails: the scalpel.

Saul Tenser offers what lies within him – he opens himself, quite literally, before his audience. Caprice, the artist, sculpts and beautifies his entrails using a module whose original function was to perform autopsies, but which, reconfigured for artistic purposes, has become "the brush." The performance they enact is not an as if: it is what it is. And it is so to the extreme of flesh vivisection: the relentless assault on that materiality which, for metaphor and the incorporeal to exist, must remain veiled.

Flesh, through its refractory nature to the Symbolic and its forclusion within those limits, returns in its Imaginary consistency, replicating the Real in a new flesh that appears to be alive – yet is composed more of the mortification of the abstracted Signifier, through algorithms, than of vitality. This contrast between flesh and metal may indicate that the algorithmically configured objects have not, as it might seem, incarnated or acquired the materiality of flesh; rather, the létouses have taken on its image, through which they commune with its refractory property to the Symbolic, coupling with it and informing it.

Tenser suffers from Accelerated Evolution Syndrome, a condition that drives his body to develop new vestigial organs with no organic function. These are the very organs Caprice tattoos while they remain inside his body, before extracting them – thus inaugurating a proliferating and unfinished series of objets a. Cronenberg reveals both dimensions of flesh, along with the transformations they might lead us toward, once unbound. A flesh that is refractory to the Signifier and informed by algorithms: it forges an alliance with technology and lends its appearance to the létouses, while revelling in its own jouissance, and of its uncontainability – neither content nor container. And another kind of flesh: one that mutates under the incidence of the Symbolic, producing organs that serve no purpose other than the auto-satisfaction of their own reproduction. In *Crimes of the Future*, biopower seeks to regulate life by controlling bodies and flesh as the final bastion of what remains colonizable. Cronenberg presents a dystopian future in which humanity has exploited the planet and its own bodies in equal measure. There, a National Organ Registry is established, under the Unit of New Vices (U.N.V.), imposing a regime of panoptic surveillance upon the flesh – preventing mutation from becoming insurrection, and denying subjects sovereignty over their jouissance, their life, and their death.

Regarding inscriptions in the flesh and their intermixture with language, Saul says:

> It takes the shape of the organ itself. In fact, in a certain way, it dominates it, remodels it. It is not just a parasite, though I suppose in some sense it is. It seems to strip the organ of meaning, appropriating the process of signification for itself, so to speak.

Has Cronenberg read Lacan? Or do both read at the level of structure?

Lang Dotrice – leader of the "subversive" group – offers Saul the corpse of his son: the first human whose organs are capable of saving humanity from contamination. The child's body is offered as a sacrifice to expose the truth the governments seek to conceal: that human transformation lies beyond their control. This body seems to embody a third alternative – one in which both dimensions of flesh are genuinely sustained. Here, the new flesh would not be that which, severed from the human body, is informed by technology while simultaneously informing still-human flesh. Nor would it be the human flesh that, in reaction to biopower's excessive control, endlessly reproduces a series of organs. Rather, it would be a flesh that mutates its own materiality through the influence of the Symbolic and is capable of surviving by incorporating the very waste produced by the being inhabiting it.

Crimes of the Future is yet another piece in the narrative David Cronenberg has been crafting for over five decades, where the idea of the New Flesh stands at the core of his stories. An invention of artistic jouissance that encodes what this journey seeks to conclude. With its folds and scars, its fluids and secretions, flesh reminds us of our vulnerability and mortality, but also of a force that refuses to be dematerialized into algorithms and bytes. Between the literal and the metaphorical; its dreams and nightmares; hardness and flexibility; autoeroticism and libidinal charge; the Real, the Symbolic, and the Imaginary; the dictate and the trace; immutability and transformation; desire and jouissance; the explicit and the enigma; the life drive and the death drive; the organic and the artificial, redemption and perdition – and between its forgetting and presentification – flesh insists, resists, and persists. Flesh bears us.

Notes

1 Translated from the original Spanish.
2 The term "forclusion" is retained from the French to preserve its Lacanian (Lacan, 1970/2012b, p. 409) specificity, rather than translating it as "foreclosure."
3 A creepypasta is a horror story or urban legend shared online. The term is a play on words combining "creepy" and "copypasta" (a block of text frequently copied and pasted). These are usually short stories that try to appear as real experiences or urban myths, and they spread primarily through social media, forums, and dedicated websites.
4 "Is the body of the Symbolic a body? No, rather it is the model of none. . . . Because one can say body: this is not a metaphor." Lacan, J. (2012). Radiophony. In *Other writings* (p. 409). Paidós. (Original work published 1970.)
5 Lacan introduces and develops the concept of "immixtion of the Other(s)" primarily in Seminar XV, "The Psychoanalytic Act" (1967–1968).
6 "Létouse" is a term Lacan introduced in Seminar XVII to refer to objects produced by science and technology. These are technological products created by science that function as new *objet a*. Lacan associates them with the lathouses (another neologism he uses for such scientific objects). They are consumer goods that proliferate on the market – a specific form of *plus-de-jouir* characteristic of capitalist discourse. This concept highlights how science produces objects that function as causes of desire. It is significant because it points to the way science and technology generate objects that take the place of the *objet a*, producing new forms of jouissance in contemporary culture.
7 In Seminar XXII, R.S.I., Lacan states that the sensitivity of the Real is writing; I therefore understand that, insofar as writing entails inscription in what we here designate as flesh, any forclusion of flesh implies a forclusion of the sensitivity of the Real – that is, the forclusion of the Real itself, as well as the forclusion of any trace.
8 "Opercive" is a neologism that combines "opera" (to operate) and "perceive." This term suggests a mode of perception that is simultaneously an operation – that is, in the very act of perceiving, an operation is being performed on what is perceived.

Bibliography

Books

Bana, M., & Galliano, A. (2021). La muerte es un lujo innecesario. Del cosmismo ruso al transhumanismo universal. In B. Groys (Ed.), *Cosmismo ruso. Tecnologias de la inmortalidad antes y despues de la Revolucion de Octubre* (pp. 27–49). Caja Negra.

CCRU. (2022). *Hyperstition*. Materia Oscura.

Descartes, R. (2009). *Meditaciones metafisicas* (V. Pena, Trans.). Alfaguara. (Original work published 1641)

Freud, S. (1979). *The interpretation of dreams* (Complete Works, Vols. IV–V). Amorrortu Editores. (Original work published 1900)

Greiner, C. (2019). *Readings of the body in Japan and its cognitive diasporas*. Zettel Editorial Agency and Abyssal Notations.

Henry, M. (2001). *Incarnation: A philosophy of flesh* (J. Teira, Trans.). Gorka Fernández & Roberto Ranz.

Husserl, E. (1997). *Ideas pertaining to a pure phenomenology and to a phenomenological philosophy. Second book: Phenomenological investigations on constitution* (A. Zirión Qujano, Trans.). UNAM. (Original work published 1952)
Huxley, J. (1957). *New bottles for new wine*. Chatto & Windus.
Lacan, J. (1984). *The seminar. Book III: The psychoses*. Paidós. (Original work published 1955–1956)
Lacan, J. (1993). *The seminar. Book II: The ego in Freud's theory and in the technique of psychoanalysis* (I. Agoff, Trans.). Paidós. (Original work published 1954–1955)
Lacan, J. (1999). *The seminar. Book V: Formations of the unconscious*. Paidós. (Original work published 1957–1958)
Lacan, J. (2006). *El seminario, libro 10: La angustia* (E. Berenguer, Trans.). Paidos. (Original work published 1962–1963).
Lacan, J. (2012a). *The seminar. Book XX: Encore* (I. Agoff, Trans.). Paidós. (Original work published 1972–1973)
Lacan, J. (2012b). *Radiophony and television. Other writings*. Paidós. (Original work published 1970)
Merleau-Ponty, M. (2010). *Lo visible y lo invisible* (E. Consigli & B. Capdevielle, Trans.). Nueva Vision. (Original work published 1964).
Parkin, S. (2021). *Death by video game*. Turner.

Unpublished Seminars

Lacan, J. (1974–1975). *The seminar. Book XXII: R.S.I.* Unpublished.

Web Articles / News Media

Ciudad Magazine. (2020, May 18). *Scandal: Football team placed sex dolls in the stands to simulate audience presence*. https://www.ciudad.com.ar/actualidad/escandalo-equipo-futbol-puso-munecas-sexuales-sus-tribunas-simular-presencia_137732/
Cronenberg, D. (Director). (2022). *Crimes of the future* [Film]. Serendipity Point Films / Argonauts Productions / Rocket Science.
El Diario.es. (2023, December 25). *Amazon updates its legal clause in case of a zombie apocalypse*. https://www.eldiario.es/rastreador/amazon-renueva-clausula-legal-apocalipsis-zombi_132_8677681.html
El Español. (2023, June 25). *Reality surpasses "Black Mirror": Creating a virtual twin of a deceased person from telegram messages*. https://www.elespanol.com/series/20230625/realidad-black-mirror-virtual-muerto-partir-telegram/772922811_0.html
Harris, O. (Director). (2013, February 11). Be right back (Season 2, Episode 1) [TV series episode]. In C. Brooker (Creator), *Black Mirror*. Channel 4.

Part 5

Who's Afraid of Artificial Intelligence?

12 A Posthumanist Take on the AI Takeover Scenario

Francesca Ferrando

I Am . . . Online, Therefore I Am

In the 21st century, a spectre is haunting humans – the spectre of technology. Technology defines the human; in palaeontological terms, for instance, the human is that animal making tools out of tools. At a substantial level, technology maintains human life: currently, a large portion of the human population would not be able to survive without electricity, infrastructures, and machines. The commercial food chain, as well as global systems of resource management, heavily relies on AI. The Colonial Pipeline cyberattack in the United States, in May 2021, and its social consequences, is an example of the possible vulnerabilities of such a strict dependency.[1] On a geological scale, the technosphere is here to stay, even after human extinction.[2] At a functional level, more and more jobs are now performed by machines, contributing to the global rise of technological unemployment. Socially speaking, virtual reality is reality. In the perception of the current youngest generation,[3] the virtual world simply exists; there is no pre-internet. Some babies are learning to say "iPad" before they can say "mom", while many children are growing up with computer-nannies in a society that is not yet realizing the physical and psychological consequences of over-exposing developing body–minds to the screen. Digital technologies are becoming entrenched with addictive behaviours, intentionally originated in the ways social media are currently being developed.[4]

Take a subway ride in any major city of technologically advanced countries, and you will see the large majority of humans glued to their phones. Where do "I" end, where does my phone begin? Can I live without the net? The eyes are on the screen, constantly, to check the news, to call grandma, or to take a picture of the moment. We live in public, immersed and often hypnotized by the gaze of techno-Medusa[5]: I am online, therefore . . . I Am. Descartes' *cogito ergo sum*[6] has turned into a self-representational mode, where individual phenomenological experiences have been disassembled and reassembled into virtual replicas: I Am . . . Being Watched. Social media

DOI: 10.4324/9781003783862-18

visibility thus becomes key to self-identity: I exist because other people see me. In the economy of social control, this pattern works both ways; you want to be seen in society, and society wants to know everything about you, because, in the Information Age, "you" are data, and your data is a precious item sold in the submerged economy of data brokers, typically without consumer agreement or acknowledgement.[7] Self-identity is constantly reconstituted in instant cyber-affinities, where your "likes" help you connect to others through similarities categorized for market research and advertising purposes. In this open frame, the border is lost; there is no "you" without the cyber gaze, and there is no cyber gaze without you. . . . Today I am watching you; and tomorrow you may be watching me, and God has always been watching us; but now that, according to Nietzsche, God is dead,[8] we need a substitute: now we have technology. Everywhere. We will never be alone again. Even if you are not watching us, you may watch that video recording of our glamorous journey to the supermarket tomorrow, one year from now, or after we die. We used to take a picture to remember the moment; now we take a picture to create a memory, and by the time we grab our phone to take a picture, that rare butterfly may be gone forever. . . . The desire to remember, and to be remembered, often marks the loss of awareness of the present moment, with extreme ramifications. Suicide videos, streamed live on Facebook, are spreading online in a psychotic twist where virtual presence (live or posthumous) is perceived as giving physical life meaning. The sacrifice of the *Carpe diem*[9] (usually translated from Latin as "Seize the day") is measured in the trading of the living moment for the (re)generation of its replicas in their cyber-gospels. As my friend wrote me when I gave birth to my child: "Now I want a picture or it did not happen!".[10] Human communication mediated by digital technology is a phenomenology of the 21st century.

AI Has Already Taken Over

The realization of artificial intelligence having already taken over should not be taken as a neutral statement, nor does this entail an uncritical acceptance of the way specific types of technological manifestations are being actualized. Instead, it is a wake-up call to be aware of where we are at – as individuals, as a society, as a species, and as a planet. We must be conscious of the narratives we are supporting. Indeed, words create worlds. The fear-based AI takeover scenario based on the division of "us" humans versus "them" (machines, robots, or AI; meaning, more generally, advanced technology) is very popular in Western countries and constantly reiterated in the narratives of mainstream media. It can be summarized in the anthropocentric tale: "we" humans may soon lose the ontological crown (or, to be clear, the dominion of the planet), so better watch out! The new war is against the supposedly evil rebellious machines, which are acting like servants, but silently robbing "us" of our planetary sovereignty. Which humans are actually at risk of being dethroned, in this ontological war, is not specified; but it should be, given that many categories of humans have not been granted any primacy in political dynamics – for instance, through technologies of social disenfranchisement, such as systemic racism and systemic sexism: these humans cannot lose the crown, since they were never accorded access to it, to begin with. To be fully aware of its socio-political implications, the human/machine dichotomy must be inscribed within the trajectory of rigid dualisms from where it stems: nature/culture, male/female, white/black, West/East, hetero/gay, and so on. Such absolute separations, generated out of the archetypal divides of self/other, us/them and right/wrong, have been historically constructed to strategically sustain specific systems of socio-political and economic domination of some humans over other (human and non-human) beings. They have caused long-lasting individual, social, and planetary traumas, and can no longer be uncritically reiterated. The dichotomy human/machine is part of these larger historical constructions and needs to be deconstructed with awareness in order to avoid perpetuating systems of oppression.

Cultural products are our current mythologies, foundational narratives in the making of the present and futures. The power of such seemingly innocent tales cannot be underestimated; the risk of self-fulfilling prophecies is real and well demonstrated.[11]

In reiterating AI as the enemy, such symbolic memes are actually creating the dreaded enemy, which may not be AI, but the human intentions behind the development of AI. Within this distorted frame, the solution to the fear of AI takeover becomes the self-fulfilling prophecy: in order to beat machines, humans must become machines. This type of narrative is clearly portrayed in the scenario suggested by Elon Musk, who, in 2016, co-founded the neurotechnology company Neuralink.[12] According to Musk, AI is a real threat; he thus calls for the need for a regulatory body that oversees the development of superintelligence.[13] A regulatory body is certainly needed at this stage of things, but, according to Musk, this is not enough. As he states, "humans risk being treated like house pets by artificial intelligence unless technology is developed that can connect brains to computers".[14] Haunted by the spectre of technology, Musk enters into the dethroning game in the name of fear. According to him, the only way to win over AI is, on same level, to become AI. The fight against the AI takeover scenario is a vital intention behind Neuralink, which is developing brain–machine interfaces to wirelessly connect humans and computers by inserting the device directly into the brain. The point here is not to downplay these types of technologies, which may be beneficial in different ways. Currently, similar devices are already being employed with significant results; for instance, deep brain stimulation is used to treat Parkinson's disease and treatment-resistant depression, among other conditions.[15] The urgent issue to tackle is the narrative of fear based on the moral imperative: become technology, or die out. Fear should never be the drive, nor the intention, of technological induction into society.

An uncritical claim of the cyborg based on fear is deeply problematic. Once biology and technology are merged in the run to win over the spectre of technology, substantial risks – connected, for instance, to the capitalistic paradigm in which they are inscribed – manifest themselves for real. Take technological surveillance, for instance, or data sovereignty and reusability. New layers of awareness are necessary in becoming cyborg during a historical time when mass surveillance is increasingly relying upon big data collection. Considering the far-reaching consequences of privacy breach and manipulation (as in the case of psychological targeting in the Facebook–Cambridge Analytica data scandal in 2018),[16] giving private companies access to such sensitive data, such as brain and neuronal activity, is a serious leap of faith. The hybrid imagery of organism and machine fills our minds, our media, and our culture. The symbol of our era is no longer human. This is the cyborg era, made up of technological connectivity instead of biological purity, as Donna Haraway predicted in the classic, A Cyborg Manifesto (1985). And still, such hybrid imagery and realities come with strings attached: they are still human-centric; they are developed within the economic paradigm of neo-capitalism, where biology turns into data and life becomes surplus[17]; they pertain to the geological era of the Anthropocene, or Capitalocene, with capital greed as a major cause of the current ecological devastation. In order to understand AI, we cannot get lost in anthropocentric fears nor in transhumanist excitements[18]; instead, we must become aware of where we are at, as individuals, as a society, as a species, and as a planet.

Aware

Technology cannot be reduced to some technical objects we are "using"; it must be seen for what it is: an ontological manifestation partaking in the existential revealing. A posthumanist perception of technology also realizes that technology is not neutral and that different types of technologies are generated out of specific societies, thus reflecting unique issues, intentions, and habits. For instance, the sexist and racist biases currently embedded in algorithms show where we are at in our social misconceptions.[19] Transformative power lies in the ways humans perceive technology. As a society, we can no longer think of technology in separation from humanity and ecology. Its material production has to be taken into consideration as well; thus, technology must be approached, more clearly, as an eco-technology[20]: from the environmental hazard of electronic waste – dramatically affecting civilians, wildlife, and lands – to the rising issue of space debris caused by satellites in orbit. We need to think about these crucial points in related and interdisciplinary ways. Technology, humanity, and ecology are deeply connected. We must be aware of our technological habits and, possibly, addictions; of our intentions and, possibly, reactions. We must be aware that fear cannot be the motivator of technological induction, and that the divide self/other is never absolute. We must be aware that technology is a reflection of where we are at as a society, and also, that it is an existential manifestation exceeding the human paradigm. Anthropocentrism will not save humanity. Humanity can only save themselves by understanding who we are: part of a planet, nets of ecological and technological emergences, and expressions of cosmic phenomena. Awareness is self-awareness. We do not have to await the advent of superintelligent AI for technology to be aware. Awareness is the mark of existence; in this sense, technology is already aware. And so, are we . . .

Acknowledgements

This chapter was originally published under an Open Access CC BY-SA - Attribution-ShareAlike license. The original publication, "Who is Afraid of Artificial Intelligence? A Posthumanist Take on the AI Takeover Scenario" was published by Noema Media & Publishing on June 29, 2022, as part of the European Commission Collection "Humanities and Artificial Intelligence", edited by Freddy Paul Grunerty. The author grants Routledge permission to use this article for inclusion in this book, including for commercial purposes, in accordance with the terms of the license. Francesca Ferrando, New York, December 22nd, 2025.

Thanks to Friedrich-Paul Grunert for inviting me to contribute to this important topic, and to Matigan King and Thomas Roby for their generous feedback. Thank you for reading this article and taking the time to intentionally envision the world we are manifesting. Peace and much appreciation to you all. License Creative Commons BY-NC-SA.

Notes

1 Sanger, D., Krauss, C., & Perlroth, N. (2021, May 8). Cyberattack forces a shutdown of a top U.S. pipeline. *New York Times*.
2 Haff, P. K. (2013). Technology as a geological phenomenon: Implications for human well-being. In C. N. Waters, J. Zalasiewicz, & M. Williams (Eds.), *A stratigraphical basis for the Anthropocene* (pp. 301–309). Geological Society.
3 Different people from different fields claim to have coined the term "Igeneration", while "Igen" is more specifically related to the work of Jean Twenge (2017).
4 Alter, A. (2018). *Irresistible: The rise of addictive technology and the business of keeping us hooked*. Penguin Books.
5 According to Greek Mythology, gaze would turn the viewers into stone.
6 This quotation is first found in part IV of his "Discourse on the Method" (1637).
7 Zuboff, S. (2019). *The age of surveillance capitalism: The fight for a human future at the new frontier of power*. Profile Books.
8 As theorized in "Thus Spoke Zarathustra" [1883–5] (1976).

9 A Latin aphorism found in Book 1 of Horace's lyric poems "Odes" (23 BCE).
10 Thanks to Carmel Vaisman for this note.
11 Biggs, M. (2013). *Prophecy, self-fulfilling/self-defeating, encyclopedia of philosophy and the social sciences* (p. 89). SAGE Publications.
12 https://neuralink.com/applications/.
13 Clifford, C. (2018, March 13). Elon Musk: "Mark my words – A.I. is far more dangerous than nukes". *CNBC News*.
14 Cuthbertson, A. (2020, July 27). Elon Musk claims AI will overtake humans "in less than five years". *The Independent*.
15 Kringelbach, M. L., Jenkinson, N., Owen, S. L. F., & Aziz Tipu, Z. (2007). Translational principles of deep brain stimulation. *Nature Reviews Neuroscience, 8*(8), 623–635.
16 Granville, K. (2018, March 19). Facebook and Cambridge Analytica: What you need to know as fallout widens. *The New York Times*.
17 Cooper, M. (2008). *Life as surplus. Biotechnology & capitalism in the neoliberal era*. University of Washington Press.
18 Ferrando, F. (2019). *Philosophical posthumanism* (pp. 35–38). Bloomsbury.
19 Garcia, M. (2016). Racist in the machine: The disturbing implications of algorithmic bias. *World Policy Journal, 33*(4), 111–117.
20 Ferrando, F. (2019). *Philosophical posthumanism* (pp. 118–119). Bloomsbury.

References

Alter, A. (2018). *Irresistible: The rise of addictive technology and the business of keeping us hooked*. Penguin Books.

Biggs, M. (2013). *Prophecy, self-fulfilling/self-defeating, encyclopedia of philosophy and the social sciences* (p. 89). SAGE Publications.

Clifford, C. (2018, March 13). Elon Musk: "Mark my words – A.I. is far more dangerous than nukes". *CNBC News*.

Cooper, M. (2008). *Life as surplus. Biotechnology & capitalism in the neoliberal era*. University of Washington Press.

Cuthbertson, A. (2020, July 27). Elon Musk claims AI will overtake humans "in less than five years". *The Independent*.

Ferrando, F. (2019). *Philosophical posthumanism*. Bloomsbury.

Garcia, M. (2016). Racist in the machine: The disturbing implications of algorithmic bias. *World Policy Journal, 33*(4), 111–117.

Granville, K. (2018, March 19). Facebook and Cambridge Analytica: What you need to know as fallout widens. *The New York Times*.

Haff, P. K. (2013). Technology as a geological phenomenon: Implications for human well-being. In C. N. Waters, J. Zalasiewicz, & M. Williams (Eds.), *A stratigraphical basis for the Anthropocene* (pp. 301–309). Geological Society.

Haraway, D. (1985). Manifesto for cyborgs: Science, technology, and socialist feminism in the 1980s. *Socialist Review, 80*, 65–108.

Kringelbach, M. L., Jenkinson, N., Owen, S. L. F., & Aziz Tipu, Z. (2007). Translational principles of deep brain stimulation. *Nature Reviews Neuroscience, 8*(8), 623–635.

Sanger, D., Krauss, C., & Perlroth, N. (2021, May 8). Cyberattack forces a shutdown of a top U.S. pipeline. *New York Times*.

Twenge, J. (2017). *iGen: Why today's super-connected kids are growing up less rebellious, more tolerant, less happy – And completely unprepared for adulthood – And what that means for the rest of us*. Atria Books.

Zuboff, S. (2019). *The age of surveillance capitalism: The fight for a human future at the new frontier of power*. Profile Books.

Index

Note: page numbers followed by an 'n' indicate a note on the corresponding page.

For Product Safety Concerns and Information please contact our EU
representative GPSR@taylorandfrancis.com
Taylor & Francis Verlag GmbH, Kaufingerstraße 24, 80331 München, Germany

www.ingramcontent.com/pod-product-compliance
Ingram Content Group UK Ltd.
Pitfield, Milton Keynes, MK11 3LW, UK
UKHW020001200926
475702UK00015B/2405
* 9 7 8 1 0 4 1 3 2 6 6 0 1 *